PAIN MANAGEMENT IN SPECIAL CIRCUMSTANCES

Edited by **Nabil A. Shallik**

Pain Management in Special Circumstances
http://dx.doi.org/10.5772/intechopen.74765
Edited by Nabil A. Shallik

Contributors

Ahmed El Geziry, Ahmed Zaghw, Mohamed Koronfel, Sara Siddiqui, Arif Valliani, Edward Podgorski, Arunbha Karmakar, Muhammad Khan, Nissar Shaikh, Shakhsanam Mirishova, Yasser Mahmoud Hammad Ali Hammad, Syed Abdul Rahman, Osama Elazzouny, Dhari Almenshid, Moustafa Rezk, Mohammed Azizuddin Azizuddin Imran, Malek Alali, Thomas Zouki, Armen Haroutunian, Abdulaziz Al-Mahrezi, Asma Al-Shidhani

Notice

First published in London, United Kingdom, 2018 by IntechOpen
IntechOpen is the global imprint of INTECHOPEN LIMITED, registered in England and Wales, registration number: 11086078, The Shard, 25th floor, 32 London Bridge Street
London, SE19SG – United Kingdom
Printed in Croatia

British Library Cataloguing-in-Publication Data
A catalogue record for this book is available from the British Library

Additional hard copies can be obtained from orders@intechopen.com

Pain Management in Special Circumstances, Edited by Nabil A. Shallik
p. cm.
Print ISBN 978-1-78923-963-8
Online ISBN 978-1-78923-964-5

For EU product safety concerns:
IN TECH d.o.o., Prolaz Marije Krucifikse Kozulić 3, 51000 Rijeka, Croatia,
info@intechopen.com or visit our website at intechopen.com.

Meet the editor

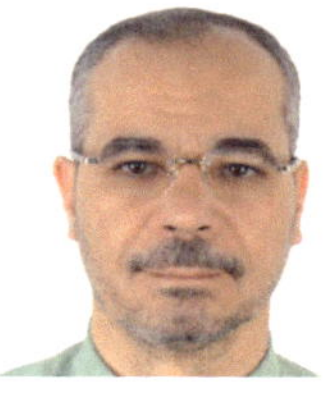

Dr. Nabil A. Shallik is a senior consultant anesthesiologist at Hamad Medical Corporation (HMC), Qatar, an Assistant Professor of clinical anesthesiology at Weill Cornell Medical College, Qatar, and an Assistant Professor of anesthesia at the Surgical Intensive Care Department, Faculty of Medicine, Tanta University, Egypt. He has several academic degrees.
Dr. Shallik is the Deputy Head of Anesthesia Department at Rumilah Hospital and Ambulatory Care Center, part of Hamad Medical Corporation in Qatar. He has published more than 35 articles in local and international peer-reviewed medical journals, including perioperative, pain and airway management publications. He is a reviewer and editorial board member for a number of international peer-reviewed medical journals and an official reviewer at the Hamad Medical Research Center.
Dr. Shallik is the principal author of many book chapters and editor of many books as well. He is a pioneer in anesthesia education and a dedicated clinical teacher; he has more than 20 years of anesthesia, intensive care, pain and perioperative medicine practice and 15 years of dedicated anesthesia teaching.
Dr. Shallik is a core faculty member of the Anesthesia Residency Program, Hamad Medical Corporation, the first ACGME-I accredited program in the Middle East. He was awarded the Award of Excellence in medical education in Qatar, best teaching material from the Fifth International Sleep Surgery Society, (5th ISSS), second place in the 3D printing competition of the 3D challenge 2017 and first place in 2018 at Texas A&M University at Qatar. He received an innovation fund from the Academic Health System in HMC for development of many projects.

Contents

Preface IX

Chapter 1 **Non-Pharmacological Pain Management 1**
Ahmed El Geziry, Yasser Toble, Fathi Al Kadhi, Muhammad Pervaiz and Mohammad Al Nobani

Chapter 2 **Pain Management for the Sickle Cell Patient 15**
Thomas Zouki, Armen Haroutunian and Tennison Malcolm

Chapter 3 **Is Chronic Post-Surgical Pain Preventable? 35**
Abdulaziz Al-Mahrezi and Asma Al-Shidhani

Chapter 4 **Acute Pain Management in Intensive Care Patients: Facts and Figures 59**
Nissar Shaikh, Saher Tahseen, Qazi Zeesan Ul Haq, Gamal Al-Ameri, Adel Ganaw, Arshed Chanda, Muhammed Zubair Labathkhan and Tariq Kazi

Chapter 5 **Pain Management for Pregnant Women in the Opioid Crisis Era 73**
Ahmed Zaghw, Mohamed Koronfel, Edward Podgorski, Sara Siddiqui, Arif Valliani, Arunabha Karmakar and Jaffar Khan

Chapter 6 **Pain Management in Patients with Impaired Kidney Function 99**
Shakhsanam Mirishova and Yasser Mahmoud Hammad Ali Hammad

Chapter 7 **Management of Acute Pain in Obese Patients with Sleep Apnea 113**
Sayed Rahman, Ahmed Zaghw, Osama Elazzouny, Dhari Almenshid, Mustafa Rezk, Mohammed Azizuddin Imran and Malek Alali

Preface

Pain control and disease management have been grown hand in hand since the dawn of life and the early practice of medicine by ancient humans.

When patients come to us with their pain, they present us with a challenging opportunity to understand them, tackle how their pain is affecting their lives, discover what is causing their pain, and finally the opportunity to prescribe medications and advise on necessary lifestyle changes to help them gain relief from their pain.

Healthcare professionals are encountered daily with different pain scenarios and they are asked to find appropriate solutions. The clinical presentation may be acute or chronic, and successful management involves an accurate diagnosis and implementation of a suitable therapy or therapies. For beginners in pain management, this can pose a significant challenge as well as for senior pain physicians.

This book will serve as a ready reference for those embarking on pain management. Its intent is not to be a heavy book that can only be stored on a bookshelf, but a pocket-sized reference that can be carried, be easily navigated, and be available whenever a conceptual gap compromises pain physicians and their ability to treat their patients.

Though this book is intended for new trainees in the field of pain management as well as senior pain practitioners, it should also be noted that it deals with pain in special circumstances and sometimes rare pain conditions that may meet the pain practice.

This book provides the latest updates on pain management in special circumstances and highlights the recent advances for evidence-based pain management.

While we did our best to prevent any misinformation of any form, we would urge our readers to inform us of any such error, including spelling or contextual errors. We also would advise that this book certainly does not replace professional or expert guidance and consultation.

We are grateful to Ms. Maja Bozicevic for her continuous help in all stages of this book. I owe my own achievements to my wife, my daughter, and my sons and I cannot thank them enough. Also, we are grateful to Professor Marco A.E. Marcus for his constant support while editing this unique book, *Pain Management in Special Circumstances*, and to all participating authors for their contributions.

Dr. Nabil A. Shallik MSc, MD
Hamad Medical Corporation
Doha, Qatar

Chapter 1

Non-Pharmacological Pain Management

Ahmed El Geziry, Yasser Toble, Fathi Al Kadhi,
Muhammad Pervaiz and Mohammad Al Nobani

Additional information is available at the end of the chapter

http://dx.doi.org/10.5772/intechopen.79689

Abstract

Non-pharmacological pain therapy refers to interventions that do not involve the use of medications to treat pain. The goals of non-pharmacological interventions are to decrease fear, distress and anxiety, and to reduce pain and provide patients with a sense of control. When deciding the most effective non-pharmacological technique, take into consideration the patient's age, developmental level, medical history and prior experiences, current degree of pain and/or anticipated pain. The advantage of non-pharmacological treatments is that they are relatively inexpensive and safe.

Keywords: pain, non-pharmacological, physical, psychological, spiritual

1. Introduction

Non-pharmacological therapies are typically categorized into

1. Physical (sensory) interventions

   Physical (sensory) interventions typically are patient-specific and inhibit nociceptive input and pain perception.

   Some measures that can reduce pain intensity and improve the patient quality of life such as massage, positioning, hot and cold treatment, transcutaneous electrical nerve stimulation (TENS), acupuncture and progressive muscle relaxation.

2. Psychological interventions

   Continuous pain may lead to development of maladaptive status and behavior that worsen day to day function, increase distress, or enhancing the experience of pain. Patients suffering pain tend to show increased vulnerability to a variety of psychiatric illnesses, including depressive and anxiety disorders, and posttraumatic stress disorder. In fact, the relationship between depression and pain is likely to be bidirectional, so that the presence of a depressive disorder has been identified as a key risk factor in the transition from acute to chronic pain.

   Most commonly used psychological interventions are: cognitive behavioral therapy, mindfulness-based stress reduction, acceptance and commitment therapy (ACT), guided imagery and biofeedback.

3. Others

   Spirituality and religion in pain management and music therapy.

2. Physical (sensory) interventions

2.1. Massage

Pain can complicate the patient condition as it can elevate stress, altering posture, and reduce one's ability to participate in daily activity [1]. It is the process of rubbing and kneading parts of the body, especially joints and muscles with hands to relieve pain and decrease tension. Massage can interrupt the patient's cycle of distress. It can increase the blood circulation as well as lymphatic circulation. Massage can also initiate an analgesic effect to the area being rubbed and decrease inflammation and edema. Moreover, it can release muscle spasms manually while increasing endogenous endorphin release, and conflicting sensory stimuli that override pain signals [2].

The process of rubbing and kneading soft tissues of the body can lead to relaxation of the tense muscles, increase blood flow to the underlying tissues and decrease pain. The exact mechanism of pain reduction in massage is still unknown; however, there are some studies and expert's hypothesis suggest that the process of massage can lead to an increase in dopamine levels which decrease pain. In addition to that, massage can lead to relaxation of the muscles tension that often arise when pain present [3].

There are many benefits of massage as it can reduce stress, promote muscle relaxation, lower blood pressure, improve circulation, help improve posture, and strengthen the body immune system. Moreover, there are some studies suggest that massage had been found to decrease pain and anxiety in many of the surgical and nonsurgical patients [3].

Massage can be beneficial in cancer patient as it can improve mood and quality of life among patients suffering from cancer. Both the massage and simple-touch groups had statistically, although not clinically, significant improvements in pain and quality of life over time despite no increases in total analgesic medication use [4]. In addition to that, there are some short-term benefits of massage which include improve psychological well-being and, in some cases, reduced severity of physical symptoms. Depression and anxiety have shown significantly improve with massage.

2.2. Positioning

Positioning is a physical intervention that includes maintaining a proper body alignment to reduce stress and anxiety, especially in children.

It helps to prevent further complications, reduces the risk for developing injuries, prevents developing bed ulcers and most importantly reduce alleviate pain. Therefore, positioning the patient correctly and re-positioning can help with the above complications [5].

Positioning can help with many patients as it can relieve muscle pain, tension and discomfort. It can improve blood circulation which in turn prevents ulcers from developing. Moreover, elevating extremities while positioning can be beneficial in decreasing pain and prevent edema as well.

2.3. Hot and cold

Several studies have shown reduction in pain, anxiety, nausea and heart rate in patients treated with active warming for pain related to mild trauma, cystitis, urolithiasis, cholelithiasis, appendicitis, colitis, and rectal trauma. This is an inexpensive and easy-to-use therapy with minimal side effects when used appropriately. Cold therapy includes applying a cool substance or device to any part of the body. Numerous studies have reported that cold treatment can increase pain threshold, decrease edema, and suppress the inflammatory process. Cold compresses may be used between 15 and 30 min time periods and up to 2–3 times per day.

Hot and cold therapy has been used for many decades and centuries to relieve pain, which includes muscle pain, joints pain, extremities pain, back pain and arthritis. Some studies show evidence that ice and heat therapies are effective and can reduce pain when compared to over the counter meds such as Paracetamol and Ibuprofen.

One study showed that "superficial heat relieves pain in a number of different ways:

1. Heat stimulates the thermo receptors in the skin and deeper tissues. This can help to reduce pain by closing the gating system in the spinal cord.
2. Heat reduces striated muscle spasm by minimizing muscle spindle excitability and reducing tension in muscle trigger points.
3. By warming joints, heat reduces the viscosity of synovial fluid, which alleviates painful stiffness during movement and increase joint range" [5].

Although through history hot and cold-water therapy is frequently used in home environment. However, these home therapies can create some complications such as burns and water leak. Nowadays, mostly in hospital setting, they use wheat-based heat packs and electrical heating pads, which are safer and give the maximum effect of analgesics [6].

2.4. Acupuncture

This has been used for around 5000 years, and it is considered one of the world's oldest arts of an empiric body healing. Basically, acupuncture works by putting the needle in specific region of the body, which stimulates the nerve. Each needle will cause no discomfort to little discomfort to the patient, but it will produce a small injury at the insertion area which will stimulate the body and the immune system to increase circulation, wound healing, pain modulation and pain analgesia [7].

The number and location of the acupuncture used by Chinese ancient times has changed by the science of modern practitioners, and nowadays they are using clinical and physical observation of the patient and the therapeutic effect of the pricking. According to Lewin (1974) "Two therapeutic modes of acupuncture are used in practice today: (1) acupuncture used for the treatment of many diseases and (2) acupuncture employed as an anesthetic procedure (a more accurate term for this would be surgical analgesia)" [8].

Acupuncture can be used to treat many conditions and studies claiming that it can be helpful with allergies, anxiety and depression, chronic back, neck, or shoulders pain, hypertension, insomnia, migraines, morning sickness, strokes and menstrual cramps. In addition to that studies suggest that it can be beneficial with cancer and multiple sclerosis patients as well [9]. The benefits of acupuncture can go beyond conditions to go far to help with relaxation and pain management as well. Acupuncture can be helpful as an analgesic effect to patients who experience pain as well [7].

2.5. Transcutaneous electrical nerve stimulation

Transcutaneous electrical nerve stimulation (TENS) is an electrical device used to treat pain. It consists of battery-powered unit and has 2–4 leads connected to sticky pads, which are positioned over the skin to cover or surround the painful area.

The TENS unit delivers a low-voltage electrical impulse to the padded surface electrodes in a series of alternating electrical current impulses.

The larger impulses are postulated to activate large myelinated fibers.

Large nerve fiber stimulation is thought to block small pain-transmitting fibers. Some experts also believe that TENS unit activates the release of natural endorphins at the pituitary level by using alternating low-540 frequency pulses.

It is thought that TENS produce analgesia by stimulating large afferent fibers. It can help those patients with chronic back pain, arthritis, and neuropathic pain. In addition, it can help patients with mild to moderate acute pain.

When the TENS unit is turned on, patient feeling a light tingling sensation over the area where the pads are placed.

The signal intensity also known as pulse width (duration of the pulse) produced from the TENS device can be adjusted, the goal being to produce paresthesia without muscle contraction. At initial use, the patient adjusts the settings to find the most comfortable effective sensation [10].

TENS is virtually side effect free, and the mechanism includes activation of descending modulation systems and blocking of sympathetic outflow.

The unit can be attached to the patient's belt for ease of use.

TENS should not be used in patients with cardiac pacemakers or a history of cardiac dysrhythmia [11].

2.6. Progressive muscle relaxation

Progressive muscle relaxation is a technique where the participant involved tightens and relaxes different muscle groups throughout the body in a progressive manner that would provoke a sense of relaxation and comfort.

There are many indications to the use of PMR, including back pain, phantom limb pain, headache and stress. PMR is a safe technique with minimal if any adverse effects have been reported.

In a double-blinded randomized clinical trial the use of PMR was found to decrease intensity of pain, tenderness of masticatory muscles and maximum opening of mouth with and without pain in patient with myofascial pain dysfunction syndrome [12].

Relaxation techniques have shown positive results for patients with chronic neck pain, tension headache, low back pain and chronic pain related to rheumatologic and non-rheumatologic chronic inflammatory disorders [13–19].

The global spine care initiative for communities with low and medium income supports the use of biofeedback and progressive muscle relaxation techniques as an initial therapy for patient without a serious pathology chronic low back pain and neck pain [20].

In a randomized controlled trial, it was found that the use of PMR in combination with guided imagery and phantom exercises were useful in reducing phantom limb pain and phantom limb sensation [21].

In an interesting study which looked into deploying relaxation techniques over the Internet was found to be effective for patient suffering from chronic headaches. Other trials are ongoing that utilizes phone applications in other conditions like chronic back pain and neck pain [14, 22].

3. Psychological interventions

3.1. Cognitive behavioral therapy

Incorporating the biopsychosocial (BPS) model to pain management by targeting cognitive responses to pain and maladaptive behavioral in addition to social and environmental factors that may play an important role in modifying reactions to pain [23]. Such therapy has shown efficacy for many physical disorders and psychiatric illnesses, as well as pain [24]. Cognitive behavioral therapy (CBT) helps to develop important set of coping skills intended to improve psychological functioning, including behavioral activation, structured relaxation exercises, recalling and scheduling of pleasurable events, dogmatic assertive communication, and behavior pacing aiming to avoid prolongation and/or exacerbation of flares of pain. CBT for pain also addresses maladaptive thoughts about pain and pain catastrophizing through formal use of cognitive restructuring.

According to recent meta-analytic studies [25], CBT for pain demonstrates small-to-medium effect sizes in a variety of domains and shows effects on pain and functioning compared to standard medical care for pain.

3.2. Mindfulness-based stress reduction

This approach aims to disconnect the link between the sensory elements of pain from the emotional and evaluative elements and enhances uncoupled awareness of both somatic and psychological sensations [26]. Because the signal of pain usually cannot be distinguished, such detachment may alter the response to pain [27].

Using mindfulness-based stress reduction strategies such as awareness and meditation, different ideas and beliefs about pain may be perceived as an unattached event rather than a sign of an underlying matter that requires lineal and possibly maladaptive reactions.

3.3. Acceptance and commitment therapy

This approach implies that thoughts do not basically have to be changed or targeted but the responses to these thoughts may be altered in a way that the resulting negative consequences are ameliorated [28]. ACT approaches can augment the sense of well-being via purposeful and nonjudgmental acknowledgment of mental events like emotions and thoughts, facilitating acceptance of such events, and enhancing the capability of the patients to sustain present and be aware of personally relevant environmental and psychological factors. Keeping this in mind, patients might be able to modify their behavior in a way that is in line with their goals and values, instead of keep focusing on immediate relief from their emotions and thoughts [27]. While conducting pain management, ACT can boost purposeful awareness and pain acceptance, hence diverting the focus on decreasing pain and its thought content and re-directing efforts trying to achieve favorable fulfilling behavior.

3.4. Biofeedback

Applied psychophysiology or better known as biofeedback is a technique in which the patient receives extra "extrinsic" information that is not based on what the patient feels, and the information should be in real time and biological in nature, that is, the use of real-time ultrasound biofeedback for patient with pelvic floor muscle dysfunction or low back pain, or the use of electromyography (EMG) in real time for patients with musculoskeletal disorders [29]. In simple words by Schawarts and Olsen, "psychophysiology involves the scientific study of the interrelation of physiological and cognitive processes" [30–32].

In a randomized clinical trial, it looked into the difference between hypnosis for chronic low back pain and hypnosis with biofeedback techniques, it showed that biofeedback with hypnosis is significantly more effective than hypnosis alone [33].

In a meta-analysis by Sielski, he found that biofeedback led to a small to medium effect when it comes to pain intensity reduction in patients with chronic back pain, also it led to reducing depression, disability, muscle tension, and improved cognitive coping in the same patients' groups [34]. Biofeedback was also used successfully in patients with juvenile rheumatoid arthritis, in a randomized clinical trial for children aged 8–13, the use of electromyography biofeedback was associated with reduced pain intensity and improved quadriceps strength [35].

3.5. Guided imagery

It is a technique in which an experienced practitioner helps a patient provoke a state of mind or mental images in the absence of that stimuli, defined by Bresler and Rossman as a range of techniques from simple visualization and direct imagery-based suggestions through metaphor and storytelling [36]. Recently, it has been increasingly explored in different medical settings, like for managing post-operative pain, fibromyalgia, low back pain or musculoskeletal-related pain.

Those images if they are vivid enough, this may elicit a physiological response, through modulations at the level of the autonomic nervous system, such effects would result in changes of the cardiovascular, respiratory, nervous, endocrine and even immune system [37]. Many randomized clinical trials have shown significant reduction in pain scores using guided imagery or hypnosis, but there is a lack of rigors high-quality studies, in a systematic review by Posadzki, he found only nine RCT with quality ranged between 1 and 3 on Jadad scale, eight of them suggested significant reduction of musculoskeletal-related pain, while one showed no significant change from the usual standard of care [38].

In another systematic review of randomized clinical trial by Posadzki, he found that 11 trails of the 15 included in his analysis showed significant reduction of non-musculoskeletal pain, while 4 trails showed no significant change from standard of care. Although the evidence remains inconclusive but simply looking at the risk to benefit ratio, we can simply conclude that benefits significantly outweigh the risk [39].

Many trials have looked into the efficacy of guided imagery and hypnosis in fibromyalgia cases, were they have shown a clinically significant benefit, moreover, a meta-analysis by Zechhave showed that combined therapy of cognitive behavioral therapy and hypnosis is superior to the use of cognitive behavioral therapy alone in patients with fibromyalgia [40].

4. Others

4.1. Spirituality and religion

In the middle ages, pain was considered a religious matter. Pain was seen as God's punishment for sins, or as evidence that an individual was possessed by demons. Spiritual counseling in such situation can be more of a priority than medical treatment [41]. Major parts of Hindu believers consider pain as a God punishment or as a result of personal actions. In Islam, it can be vindictive or Allah's willingness. A common Buddhist belief is that suffering is the price of attachment [42]. Spiritual and religious beliefs are important in many individuals' lives.

However, religious and spirituality are not the same. These beliefs can influence lifestyle, attitudes, and feelings about life, pain, and death. Spiritual and religious beliefs are important in many individuals' lives. However, religious and spirituality are not the same. These beliefs can influence lifestyle, attitudes, and feelings about life, pain, and death. Spiritual beliefs often place a greater significance at the time of illness than any other time in a person's life.

Both religious and spiritual beliefs help some people accept their own illness and help explain illness for others. Religion can supply the client, the family, and health professionals with a sense of strength, security, and faith during a time of need [41, 43].

Pain is an extremely complex phenomenon that involves multiple cascades of behavioral responses, thoughts, and emotions. A lot of non-physiologic factors such as psychological, familial and societal attitudes, life stressors, and cultural, spiritual and religious beliefs contribute significantly how the individuals experience and respond to pain. Emotional distress specifically depression and anxiety plays a vital role in pain experience. Numerous studies have demonstrated that individuals having pain perhaps report more severe pain and disability, if they have anxiety, depression or both. Interestingly, it has been found that fear of pain can cause more disability than that has been already caused by pain itself. There is a cyclical pattern of chronic pain leading to depression and depression causing an increase in chronic pain, creating a mutually reinforcing relationship [44, 45].

Since pain experienced in the context of biopsychosocial-spiritual system model (BPSSM), it should be understood that individuals' capacities to cope, tolerate, and accept disease and pain entail multiple levels of experience and thought. BPSSM suggests that illness disrupts the biological, interpersonal, and spiritual relationships unique to the individual. The BPSSM recognizes the potential impact of spiritual and religious variables that may increase or decrease experience of illness.

Spiritual interventions may differ depending on culture background. Generally, prayer is one of the most common daily spiritual activities, which can take variety of forms including gratitude, admission and confession, intercessory prayer or silent communion. The ultimate goal is to become more close to and loved one for God. Pain is often referenced in the context of people's relationships with God. God is responsible for wellbeing and health; therefore, spiritual beliefs are considered one of the most effective ways that influence healing. Individuals suffering pain may practice varieties of spiritual and religious activities including prayer and seeking specialized spiritual support, to cope more effectively with their pain [46]. Patients with chronic pain with a variety of conditions (e.g., musculoskeletal pain, cancer, or sickle cell) usually report that religiousness and spirituality are important in their lives [47].

4.2. Music therapy

Music has been used since ancient times to enhance wellbeing and reduce pain and suffering. Playing music for patients during or after surgery helps reduce pain and use of morphine and other sedatives, anxiolytics, and analgesics [48, 49].

Many randomized controlled studies adopting music therapy for subjects undergoing colonoscopy or sigmoidoscopy have found in comparison with the control group, those who listened to music reported a significant lower pain scores, less sedation and shorter examination times [50–52].

During labor, music has been shown to reduce women perceptions of and responses to pain. The same findings have been reported in premature infants as well as other categories of individuals living with chronic pain [53, 54]. Women during labor who enjoyed listening to slow soft music experienced less distress attributed to pain and repotted music as a helpful and effective tool in pain control [54]. Elderly patients with chronic osteoarthritis who listened to music daily for twenty minutes for couple of weeks reported decreased pain levels as compared to a control group [55]. Cancer survivors reported moderate pain relief upon listening to music, and in many cancer centers, music is offered as an adjunctive therapy [56, 57].

One study has been designed to evaluate the effects of including music therapy on pain report, nausea, in addition to the time to engraftment for patients undergoing bone marrow transplant. Among such extremely ill individuals, those who received music therapy alongside with relaxation imagery experienced lower pain scales and less nausea. Moreover, they had faster engraftment [58].

5. Conclusion

The role of non-pharmacological approaches to pain management is evolving, and some non-pharmacological and complementary therapies have an increasingly important contribution to make to holistic patient care alongside analgesics.

Generally, these approaches are relatively inexpensive with high safety profile and low side effects.

There is evidence to support the use of patient education, cognitive behavioral therapy (CBT), relaxation, music, and other modalities. These therapies should be taken into consideration to help and support the standard pharmacological treatment in pain management. While medical drugs are essentially being used for treating the somatic (physiological and emotional) dimension of the pain, non-pharmacological therapies aim to treat the cognitive, affective, behavioral and socio-cultural dimensions of the pain.

These therapies can treat the pain as adjuvant or complementary at middle level and severe pain experiences.

Non-pharmacological approaches help to

- Increase the individual ability to control feeling.
- Reduce the feeling of weakness.
- Enhance the functional capacity and activity level.
- Reduces anxiety and stress.
- Decrease the pain behavior and focused pain level.
- Decrease the dosage of analgesic drugs, subsequently decreasing the well-known side effects of these drugs.

For this reason, research on non-pharmacological approaches to pain management is very important, so that patients are provided with information that ensures them the most effective options for treating their pain.

Author details

Ahmed El Geziry*, Yasser Toble, Fathi Al Kadhi, Muhammad Pervaiz and Mohammad Al Nobani

*Address all correspondence to: ageziery@hamad.qa

Department of Anaesthesia, ICU and Perioperative Medicine, Hamad Medical Corporation, Doha, Qatar

References

[1] Thompson DL. Massage, movement & mindfulness. Massage & Bodywork. 2016;**31**(5): 88-97

[2] Kutner JS, Smith MC, Corbin L, Hemphill L, Benton K, Mellis BK, et al. Massage therapy versus simple touch to improve pain and mood in patients with advanced cancer: A randomized trial. Annals of Internal Medicine. 2008;**149**(6):369-I38

[3] Ward CW. Non-pharmacologic methods of postoperative pain management. MedSurg Matters. 2016;**25**(1):9-10

[4] Rozet I, Vavilala MS. Risks and benefits of patient positioning during neurosurgical care. Anesthesiology Clinics. 2007;**25**(3):631-653

[5] Chandler A, Preece J, Lister S. Using heat therapy for pain management (clinical practice). Nursing Standard. 2002;**17**(9):40+. Available from: http://link.galegroup.com.ezproxy.lib.ucalgary.ca/apps/doc/A94820820/AONE?u=ucalgary&sid=AONE&xid=8ce9c9ba

[6] Top 6 ways to use hot and cold therapy in your practice. Massage Magazine. 2018;(261):26-27

[7] White A, Editorial Board of Acupuncture in Medicine. Western medical acupuncture: A definition. Acupuncture in Medicine. 2009;**27**(1):33

[8] Lewin AJ. Acupuncture and its role in modern medicine. Western Journal of Medicine. 1974;**120**(1):27

[9] Richardson PH, Vincent C. Acupuncture for the treatment of pain: A review of evaluative research. Pain. 1986

[10] Stannard C, Booth S. Pain. 2nd ed. Sydney, Torronto: Elsevier Churchill Livingstone; 2004

[11] Hoppenfeld JD. Multi modal approach to pain treatment. In: Fundamentals of Pain Medicine. Philadelphia: Wolters Kluwer Health; 2014. pp. 2-275

[12] Beitollahi JM, Sahebjamie M, Manavi A, Farrokhnia T, Golestan B. Effect of progressive muscle relaxation therapy on improving signs and symptoms of patients with myofacial pain dysfunction syndrome. The Journal of Dental Medicine. 2009;**21**(4):249-254. Available from: https://doaj.org/article/b2de84d7192c4bf69fd92747cc9a9b72#? [Accessed: 27-04-2018]

[13] Arena JG, Hightower NE, Chong GC. Relaxation therapy for tension headache in the elderly: A prospective study. Psychology and Aging. 1988;**3**(1):96-98. DOI: 10.1037/0882-7974.3.1.96

[14] Devineni T, Blanchard EB. A randomized controlled trial of an internet-based treatment for chronic headache. Behaviour Research and Therapy. 2005;**43**(3):277-292. DOI: 10.1016/j.brat.2004.01.008

[15] Greco CM, Rudy TE, Manzi S. Effects of a stress-reduction program on psychological function, pain, and physical function of systemic lupus erythematosus patients: A randomized controlled trial. Arthritis Care & Research (Hoboken). 2004;**51**(4):625-634. DOI: 10.1002/art.20533

[16] Flor H, Birbaumer N. Comparison of the efficacy of electromyographic biofeedback, cognitive-behavioral therapy, and conservative medical interventions in the treatment of chronic musculoskeletal pain. Journal of Consulting and Clinical Psychology. 1993;**61**(4):653-658. DOI: 10.1037/0022-006X.61.4.653

[17] Malone MD, Strube MJ. Meta-analysis of non-medical treatments for chronic pain. Pain. 1988;**34**(3):231-244. DOI: 10.1016/0304-3959(88)90118-2

[18] Astin JA. Mind–body therapies for the management of pain. The Clinical Journal of Pain. 2004;**20**(1):27-32. DOI: 10.1097/00002508-200401000-00006

[19] Metikaridis DT, Hadjipavlou A, Artemiadis A, Chrousos GP, Darviri C. Effect of a stress management program on subjects with neck pain: A pilot randomized controlled trial. Journal of Back and Musculoskeletal Rehabilitation. 2016;**30**(1):23-33. DOI: 10.3233/BMR-160709

[20] Chou R, Côté P, Randhawa K, et al. The global spine care initiative: Applying evidence-based guidelines on the non-invasive management of back and neck pain to low- and middle-income communities. European Spine Journal. 2018. DOI: 10.1007/s00586-017-5433-8

[21] Brunelli S, Morone G, Iosa M, et al. Efficacy of progressive muscle relaxation, mental imagery, and phantom exercise training on phantom limb: A randomized controlled trial. Archives of Physical Medicine and Rehabilitation. 2015;**96**:181-187. DOI: 10.1016/j.apmr.2014.09.035

[22] Blödt S, Pach D, Roll S, Witt CM. Effectiveness of app-based relaxation for patients with chronic low back pain (relaxback) and chronic neck pain (relaxneck): Study protocol for two randomized pragmatic trials. Trials. 2014;**15**(1):490. DOI: 10.1186/1745-6215-15-490

[23] Kato K, Sullivan PF, Evengård B, Pedersen NL. Chronic widespread pain and its comorbidities: A population-based study. Archives of Internal Medicine. 2006;**166**(15):1649-1654. [PubMed]

[24] Richardson LP, Russo JE, Katon W, et al. Mental health disorders and long-term opioid use among adolescents and young adults with chronic pain. The Journal of Adolescent Health. 2012;**50**(6):553-558. [PMC free article][PubMed]

[25] Hayes SC, Luoma JB, Bond FW, Masuda A, Lillis J. Acceptance and commitment therapy: Model, processes and outcomes. Behaviour Research and Therapy. 2006;**44**(1):1-25. [PubMed]

[26] Fordyce WE. Behavioral Methods for Chronic Pain and Illness. St Louis, MO: Mosby; 1976. p. 1

[27] Gatzounis R, Schrooten MG, Crombez G, Vlaeyen JW. Operant learning theory in pain and chronic pain rehabilitation. Current Pain and Headache Reports. 2012;**16**(2):117-126. [PubMed]

[28] Day MA, Thorn BE, Burns JW. The continuing evolution of biopsychosocial interventions for chronic pain. Journal of Cognitive Psychotherapy. 2012;**26**(2):114-129

[29] Giggins OM, Persson UMC, Caulfield B. Biofeedback in rehabilitation. Journal of Neuroengineering and Rehabilitation. 2013;**10**(1). DOI: 10.1186/1743-0003-10-60

[30] Hubbard D. Brief comments on the proposed definition of applied psychophysiology. Applied Psychophysiology and Biofeedback. 1999;**24**(1):41. DOI: 10.1023/A:1022842930241

[31] Schwartz MS. What is applied psychophysiology? Toward a definition. Applied Psychophysiology and Biofeedback. 1999. DOI: 10.1023/A:1022874409768

[32] Striefel S. Is the working definition of applied psychophysiology proposed by Schwartz too narrow/restrictive? Applied Psychophysiology and Biofeedback. 1999;**24**(1):11-19. DOI: 10.1023/A:1022826526606

[33] Tan G, Rintala DH, Jensen MP, Fukui T, Smith D, Williams W. A randomized controlled trial of hypnosis compared with biofeedback for adults with chronic low back pain. European Journal of Pain. 2015;**19**(2):271-280. DOI: 10.1002/ejp.545

[34] Sielski R, Rief W, Glombiewski JA. Efficacy of biofeedback in chronic back pain: A meta-analysis. International Journal of Behavioral Medicine. 2017;**24**(1):25-41. DOI: 10.1007/s12529-016-9572-9

[35] Effect of Electromyographic Biofeedback Training on Pain, Quadriceps Muscle Strength, and Functional Ability in Juvenile Rheumatoid Arthritis. 2016;**95**(12):921-930. DOI:10.1097/PHM.0000000000000524

[36] Utay J, Miller M. Journal of Instructional Psychology. 2006;**33** [V-U Pub. Co.]. Available from: https://www.questia.com/library/journal/1G1-144014458/guided-imagery-as-an-effective-therapeutic-technique [Accessed: 27-04-2018]

[37] Waldman Steven D. Pain Management. 2nd ed. Philadilphia, PA: Elsevier; 2011

[38] Posadzki P, Ernst E. Guided imagery for musculoskeletal pain. The Clinical Journal of Pain. 2011;**27**(7):648-653. DOI: 10.1097/AJP.0b013e31821124a5

[39] Posadzki P, Lewandowski W, Terry R, Ernst E, Stearns A. Guided imagery for non-musculoskeletal pain: A systematic review of randomized clinical trials. Journal of Pain and Symptom Management. 2012;**44**(1):95-104. DOI: 10.1016/j.jpainsymman.2011.07.014

[40] Zech N, Hansen E, Bernardy K, Häuser W. Efficacy, acceptability and safety of guided imagery/hypnosis in fibromyalgia—A systematic review and meta-analysis of randomized controlled trials. European Journal of Pain. 2017;**21**(2):217-227. DOI: 10.1002/ejp.933

[41] White L, Duncan G. Medical Surgical Nursing: An Integrated Approach. 2nd ed. New York: Delmar Thomson Learning; 2002

[42] Solimine MA. Spirituality. In: Hoeman SP, editor. Rehabilitation Nursing Process, Application and Outcomes. 3rd ed. St Louis: Mosby Corporation; 2002

[43] Cusick J. Spirituality and voluntary pain. APS Bulletin. 2003. Available from: http://www.ampainsoc.org/pub/bulletin/sep03/path1.htm [Accessed: 18-08-2005]

[44] Eccleston C. Role of psychology in pain management. British Journal of Anaesthesia. 2001;**87**:144-152. [PubMed]

[45] Means-Christensen AJ, Roy-Byrne PP, Sherbourne CD, et al. Relationships among pain, anxiety, and depression in primary care. Depression and Anxiety. 2008;**25**:593-600. [PubMed]

[46] Unruch A. Spirituality, religion, and pain. The Canadian Journal of Nursing Research. 2007;**39**:66-86. [PubMed]

[47] Wachholtz AB, Pearce MJ. Does spirituality as a coping mechanism help or hinder coping with chronic pain? Current Pain and Headache Reports. 2009;**13**:127-132. [PubMed]

[48] Koch ME, Kain ZN, Ayoub C, et al. The sedative and analgesic sparing effect of music. Anesthesiology. 1998;**89**:300-306

[49] Nilsson U, Rawal N, Unosson M. A comparison of intra-operative or postoperative exposure to music: A controlled trial of the effects on postoperative pain. Anaesthesia. 2003;**58**:699-703

[50] Schiemann U, Gross M, Reuter R, et al. Improved procedure of colonoscopy under accompanying music therapy. European Journal of Medical Research. 2002;**7**:131-134

[51] Smolen D, Topp R, Singer L. The effect of self-selected music during colonoscopy on anxiety, heart rate, and blood pressure. Applied Nursing Research. 2002;**15**:126-136

[52] Uedo N, Ishikawa H, Morimoto K, et al. Reduction in salivary cortisol level by music therapy during colonoscopic examination. Hepato-Gastroenterology. 2004;**51**:451-453

[53] Butt ML, Kisilevsky BS. Music modulates behaviour of premature infants following heel lance. The Canadian Journal of Nursing Research. 2000;**31**:17-39

[54] Joyce BA, Keck JF, Gerkensmeyer J. Evaluation of pain management interventions for neonatal circumcision pain. Journal of Pediatric Health Care. 2001;**15**:105-114

[55] McCaffrey R, Freeman E. Effect of music on chronic osteoarthritis pain in older people. Journal of Advanced Nursing. 2003;**44**:517-524

[56] Beck SL. The therapeutic use of music for cancer-related pain. Oncology Nursing Forum. 1991;**18**:1327-1337

[57] Standley JM, Hanser SB. Music therapy research and applications in pediatric oncology treatment. Journal of Pediatric Oncology Nursing. 1995;**12**:3-10

[58] Sahler O, Hunter B, Liesveld JL. The effect of using music therapy with relaxation imagery in the management of patients undergoing bone marrow transplantation: A pilot feasibility study. Alternative Therapies in Health and Medicine. 2003;**9**:70-74

Chapter 2

Pain Management for the Sickle Cell Patient

Thomas Zouki, Armen Haroutunian and
Tennison Malcolm

Additional information is available at the end of the chapter

http://dx.doi.org/10.5772/intechopen.79495

Abstract

Sickle cell disease (SCD) is a condition very common in the United States of America and its most common presenting symptom is pain related to vaso-occlusive events (VOE). The cost associated with healthcare for the sickle cell population exceeds 1 billion $USD yearly, and the majority of this cost is associated with admission related to vaso-occlusive events. With the increase longevity of patients with SCD, due to new therapies and vaccination against common infection related to SCD, the prevalence of older individuals experiencing VOE will likely increase. The psychological impact inflicted on patients with SCD can further complicate adequate care of patients experiencing acute or chronic pain and the latter must be taken into consideration when planning an optimal treatment regimen. This chapter reviews the short- and long-term management options of pain related to VOE, their limitations as well proposed regimen that could pave the way for the future of pain management of SCD.

Keywords: sickle cell anemia, sickle cell pain, sickle cell crises, sickle cell disease, vaso-occlusive event, sickle cell pain management, pain management

1. Introduction

Sickle cell disease (SCD) is a term used for a collective group of autosomal recessive disorders involving the abnormal structure of hemoglobin where both alleles of the beta chain of hemoglobin gene are affected, and at least one of them being affected by a sickle cell mutation. This mutation results from a single nucleotide change (GAT → GTT) in the sixth codon of the first exon of the beta-globin gene, resulting in the substitution of glutamic acid to valine (HbS) [1]. When an individual inherits two sickle cell genes (one from each parent, Hb S/S), he or she is affected with sickle cell anemia. The Hb S/S mutation is the most common form of SCD, it accounts for 60–70% of SCD in the United States. Other forms result from a coinheritance of an HbS allele with another abnormal β-globin chain, HbC (Hb S/C) and from a β-thalassemia (Hb S/β^+, Hb S/β^0) being the most common among others. The mutation results in a beta chain of the hemoglobin molecule that is more hydrophobic compared to its normal counterpart (HbB) and is prone to polymerization during episodes of lower oxygen tension, hypothermia or many other stressors. A deoxygenated hemoglobin B (HbB) of patients with SCD will aggregate along its molecular axis leading to distortion of the cell membrane and giving it a sickle shape appearance. A hallmark of sickle cell disease is intermittent vaso-occlusive events (VOE) and chronic hemolytic anemia. VOE in acute and chronic pain as well as organ damage most notably to the bones, spleen, liver, brain, lungs, kidneys and joints [2].

SCD is a disease that is mostly present in persons of African, Mediterranean, Middle Eastern and Indian ancestry but has been found in individuals of any ethnic background. The prevalence of sickle cell trait, among African Americans in the United States, is 10%, or 3.5 million people, leading to the incidence of SCD among this ethnic group of approximately 1 in 365 live births. More than 100,000 individuals in the United States are estimated to suffer from SCD. In the United Kingdom, the prevalence is about 12,500 people. Globally, it is estimated that about 5–7% of the world's population are carriers of the mutant hemoglobin gene [3, 4], most of which residing on the African continent. As a matter of fact, about 15 million Africans are affected by SCD, more than all other continents combined. And about 200–300,000 affected births per year occur on the African continent [4, 5], accounting for more than 75% of the SCD newborns worldwide. Globally, SCD is one the four most common autosomal recessive diseases along with cystic fibrosis, thalassemia and Tay-Sachs.

Although in some areas of the world, such as Western African countries, where new treatment modalities are not as widely accessible, SCD accounts for as many as 16% of deaths in children under 5 years old, the death rate has remarkably been reduced in the United States in recent times. In fact, many children did not live to adulthood about half a century ago. With the emergence of hydroxyurea, new born screening, newer and better antibiotics as well as the introduction of the pneumococcal vaccine, the lifespan for sickle cell individuals in the United States has increased substantially to 48 years old for female and 42 years old for male. As a matter of fact, the median survival age of patients with SCD living between 1910 and 1950 was below 20 years of age [6]. By 1980, 50% of children survived beyond 20 years of age; and by 2009, 85% of SCD affect patients did. In England, the trend for hospital admissions related to SCD has been on the rise; from 2001/2002 to 2009/2010, admissions with a diagnosis of SCD have risen by more than 50%.

The management of SCD is complex and multidisciplinary. Supportive management includes regular follow-ups with the healthcare providers, adequate diet and sleep. Symptomatic management targets symptoms of the disease and include blood transfusions, pain management, antibiotics for infections among many other possible treatments. Preventive managements include vaccinations, avoidance of stressors that triggers crisis, hydroxyurea treatment, transfusion, etc. Abortive therapy is the attempt at preventing painful crisis from getting worse and leading to other complications. They include nitrous oxide and anti-adhesion factors. The ultimate goal is curative therapy, which can arise from stem cell transplantation, and gene therapy in the future. This chapter focuses solely on the pain management of patients with SCD and is divided into acute pain, chronic pain and neuropathic pain.

http://dx.doi.org/10.5772/intechopen.79495

2. Pathogenesis of sickle cell pain

Sickle cell related pain is classified into three categories: acute pain, chronic pain and neuropathic pain [7]. Acute pain is, by far, the most commonly encountered type of pain by healthcare providers and is the precursor of chronic and neuropathic pain. The pathophysiology of sickle cell pain is still not completely understood but is thought to be initiated by stress/deoxygenation leading to the polymerization of sickle Hb in the red blood cells (RBC) inside the micro and macro-vasculature. This causes the RBC to lose its deformability and adhere to together on the vascular endothelium that in turn gets activated. The latter participates in the recruitment of white blood cells (WBC), which further accentuates the existing vascular occlusion and facilitates tissue ischemia and damage. The activation of endothelial cells along with the tissue damage provokes the release of inflammatory mediators (including arachidonic acid, histamines, bradykinin, H+, K+, cytokines, serotonin, substance P, leukotrienes among others) [8, 9]. The combination of tissue damage and the resulting secondary inflammatory process generated is thought to be the cornerstone of the pain perceived during VOE. They convert chemical and mechanical energy into electrochemical impulse. The release of interleukin-1 activates the cyclo-oxygenase (COX) system that in turns converts arachidonic acid into prostaglandins E2 and I2. This inflammatory soup created interacts to permit and facilitate the transduction and transmission of the painful stimuli from the periphery the central nervous system via the nerve endings, spinal cord and the thalamus. Some of the mediators (Substance P and bradykinin) also cause vasodilatation and extravasation of fluid leading to focal edema and tenderness in the affected areas.

The peripheral nociceptors involved in the painful cascade send their signals via fast acting A-delta and slow acting C fibers to the dorsal horn of the spinal cord by means of the dorsal root ganglion. From the dorsal horn of the spinal cord, the pain signals travel contralaterally through the spinothalamic tract to the thalamus that in turn has multiple interconnections with other systems such as the limbic system (mediator of memory and emotion), the reward system (mediator of pleasure and addiction) and the glia. The signals are then either facilitated or suppressed at the level of the spinal cord by different modulators. The N-methyl-D-aspartate (NMDA) receptor is probably the most important receptor involved in the facilitation of pain transmission. Other important modulators include endogenous endorphins, serotonin and norepinephrine. With knowledge of the implicated factors involved in sickle cell pain, better management can be made targeting the involved transmitters, receptors and modulators.

3. Acute pain: the vaso-occlusive event

The vaso-occlusive event (VOE) is the most common cause of morbidity in the patients with SCD [10]. VOE also account for the most common cause of hospital admissions and missed school days. Some data report that up to 95% of hospital admissions related to SCD are for acute painful crises [11, 12]. Multicellular aggregates leading to blood flow obstruction in small blood vessels, depriving downstream tissues of oxygen and nutrient constitute the painful pathway of VOE, which was described earlier in this chapter. Although VOE-related pain can affect any part of the body and often cause generalized pain, it more commonly presents as pain in the extremities in the pediatric population, as opposed to being more commonly seen as headache, chest pain, abdominal and back pain in older individuals [13]. The average duration of an acute pain crisis, based on hospital length of stay, is about 7 days [7]. Fever and leukocytosis typically accompany the patient's presentation and the extent of WBC tends to correlate with the degree of pain [14, 15]. Also, the higher the level of Hb and hematocrit is, the more likely it is that a VOE will occur [9]. Even if leukocytosis associated with VOE does not necessarily signify an infectious process, careful evaluation should be undertaken, as these individuals are highly susceptible to pathogens. A careful and thorough history and physical examination should be undertaken. Inquiring about the onset, location, radiation, quality, relieving and aggravating factors associated with the current painful episode, any differences between the current episode and previous episodes, the presence of fever, transfusion history, medications, baseline hemoglobin level, and a thorough physical exam can assist in making a more definite diagnosis. Any atypical presentation should prompt further investigation (**Table 1**). The triggers of VOE can be physical, psychological, physiological and environmental among many. At any age group, a painful crisis typically begins with sudden onset of pain.

Although most individuals with SCD presenting to the healthcare professional with VOE will exhibit different types complains as far as onset, location, quality and intensity of their pain, the painful crisis will typical last between 7 and 10 days and can be described as possessing four different phases: A prodromal phase, initial phase, established phase and resolving phase [16–18]. A prodromal phase lasts 1–2 days and consists of aches, numbness or paresthesia in the area that will subsequently become painful. Physical signs of the prodromal phase include loss of usual appearance of the eyes (loss of luster or yellowing of the eyes). Laboratory values are significant for a decrease in erythrocyte deformability and increase density of erythrocytes. The second phase, initial phase, also lasting 1–2 days, is characterized by an increase in pain level and laboratory findings such as decreased RBC deformability, increase in the number of dense cells, red cell distribution width (RDW), reticulocytosis, leukocytosis, and relative

1. Detailed history:
    - Pain: onset, location, radiation, quality, frequency, progressiveness, alleviating and aggravating factors, home medications.
    - Presence of fever
    - Transfusion history
    - Baseline hemoglobin
    - Associated factors (Cough and respiratory symptoms, GI symptoms, neurological changes)
2. Thorough physical exam
    - Body temperature
    - Areas of tenderness
    - Cardiac, pulmonary, skin, CNS, abdominal
3. Laboratory results (BMP, CBC)
4. Radiologic imaging based on history and physical (i.e., Abdominal CT for abnormal abdominal pain, Head CT if any CNS manifestation present)
5. Initiate pain management algorithm (**Figure 1**) after serious complications rules out (stroke, acute chest syndrome, splenic sequestration, pneumococcal sepsis, priapism)

Table 1. Primary investigation upon initial presentation of a SCD patient in pain.

thrombocytopenia. The third phase, the established phase, is when the pain level is at its peak. The patient will show signs of frustration, depression, will tend to complain about hospital staff due to lack of appropriate treatment. Physical exam will show an elevated temperature, signs of inflammation, joint effusions. Laboratory signs will consist of elevated WBC, decreased Hb, and elevated reticulocyte count, elevated LDH, CPK and CRP. This phase is the longest for an average of about 4–5 days. The fourth and final phase, lasting 3 days on average, is the resolving phase; patients start showing signs of decreasing pain, RBC deformability increases, as well as fibrinogen, orosomucoid, ESR, platelets and plasma viscosity. The blood level of sickled RBC is decreased during the final phase. The increase in plasma viscosity leads to a hypercoagulable state that becomes a culprit for recurrence of another painful crisis. In fact, about 16% of hospital admissions because of VOE get readmitted with recurrence within 1 week of discharge [11, 19]. The reasons for readmissions include, but not limited to, withdrawal syndrome, premature discharge, inadequate pain management during hospital admission, development of tolerance to opioid medications, opioid-induced hyperalgesia (OIH). Analysis of children admitted to hospitals with VOE show that patients typically show a blunted response to pain relief after the fourth to sixth day of admission [20]. The reason for this phenomenon is unknown but could be related to OIH, tolerance or provider inexperience with prolonged VOE pain. This subset of patients is more likely to return to the hospital and get readmitted. Special attention should be paid to readmitted patient since these tend a have a higher morbidity and mortality rate. Also, care should be taken not to under treat patients in the resolving phase of the VOE; Even if the pain seems to subside during this phase, it is important to continue aggressive pain management, provide patients with appropriate discharge instructions to avoid overdose or withdrawal after discharge, arrange for appropriate follow-up.

This table points out important factors to consider when doing a primary investigation of a SCD patient presenting to the ED in pain. It is important to perform a full assessment of the patient to rule out any serious adverse events that are commonly associated with SCD.

3.1. Treatment of acute sickle cell pain

The first time SCD was recognized as its own disease was in 1910 when a medical resident observed the sickle appearing cell under a microscope [21]. Since then, many more discoveries about the disease were made, and its treatment still remains a dynamic process with changes constantly occurring. The therapeutic research initially consisted of finding ways to prevent the blockage of small blood vessels by the sickles shape RBC [22]. It was not until the 1960s that pain was recognized as a major symptom in SCD. Among the first pharmacological approaches used to treat it figured papaverine and acetaminophen [23]. It was not until later that opioid medications were used for the treatment of SCD and now represents the cornerstone of treatment for acute painful crisis. Appropriate treatment of VOE crisis is crucial since the consequences associated with the latter are many. Those involve acute chest syndrome in about 50% of VOE-related hospitalization, acute multi-organ failure and sudden death [24–26]. Aborting the acute painful episode at the prodromal phase could potentially prevent or minimize tissue damage [16]. A wide range of treatment modalities exists for the treatment of acute sickle cell pain. Nonpharmacological approaches such as acupuncture, heat, ice, relaxation techniques and hypnosis but are not covered in detail in this chapter [9, 27–30]. Pharmacological approaches for the treatment of VOE around the globe consist predominantly of opioid analgesic including full agonists, partial agonists, mixed agonists-antagonists, antagonists but also include opioid adjuvants as well as nonopioid analgesics such NSAIDs, acetaminophen and other adjuvants [9]. As previously mentioned, VOE is the most common presentation (up to 90%) of patients with SCD to the healthcare facilities (i.e., Emergency Department). The first step in management focuses on immediate pain control with fluids and analgesics as evidence exists demonstrating that rapid and efficient control of acute pain related to VOE reduces pain scores, length of hospital stay, improve patient satisfaction [28, 31], reduce hospitalization in patients with SCD and also a decrease in the development of chronic pain syndromes, which is commonly seen in the sickle cell population [9, 32].

However, managing the pain could be more difficult than anticipated by the healthcare provider, as the SCD patient's pain management differs from that of the rest of the population. Indeed, the patient with sickle cell disease tends to be more tolerant to opioid medications then the rest of the population due to chronic administration, VOE pain can appear out of proportion for most providers and necessitates higher doses of narcotics which most emergency department providers are not accustom to administer. This underlines the reason why most patients with sickle cell disease report that their pain is undertreated in the emergency department and that the providers lack understanding and compassion [9, 33–38]. Additionally, VOE-related pain more exaggerated than expected, every patient possesses his own unique sensation, perception and expression of pain.

Indicators of adequate VOE management consist, but not limited to, admission to the hospital (indicates poor pain control in the ED), readmission to the hospital (indicator that pain was not well controlled during hospital stay), length of stay (indicator of effective pain management during hospital stay), pain intensity felt during ED visit or hospitalization (different pain measurement assessment available), patient and parents satisfaction, increase or decrease in VOE/SCD-related complications (**Table 2**).

The indicators of an effective treatment of SCD patients during their visit to the ED or admission to the hospital are shown here. Signs of ineffective treatment are admission from the ED to the hospital, readmission to the hospital after discharge, increased length of stay in the ED or the hospital, elevated pain assessment score, poor patient and/or parent satisfaction.

Facilities that have taken into account these indicators of effective VOE pain management have demonstrated benefice in rapid treatment of patients presenting to their healthcare facility with VOE with an individualized plan for each patient. An individualized plan results in decreased hospital admissions, readmissions, length of ED and hospitalization, substantial decrease in pain scores, increased patient and parent satisfaction. Although no single plan or approach is perfect for all patients, there are different algorithms that are available to the healthcare provider that serve as helpful guide for the patient presenting with VOE. Using an algorithm has shown to be simple, cost-effective and beneficial for the patient's generalized well-being. Institutions that commonly encounter patients with VOE are encouraged to either follow an existing effective algorithm or create their own. Every patient presenting to the healthcare provider with VOE-related pain would require his or her own individualized treatment plan [39]. Our preferred algorithm is inspired by the American Pain Society and is detailed in the following paragraph.

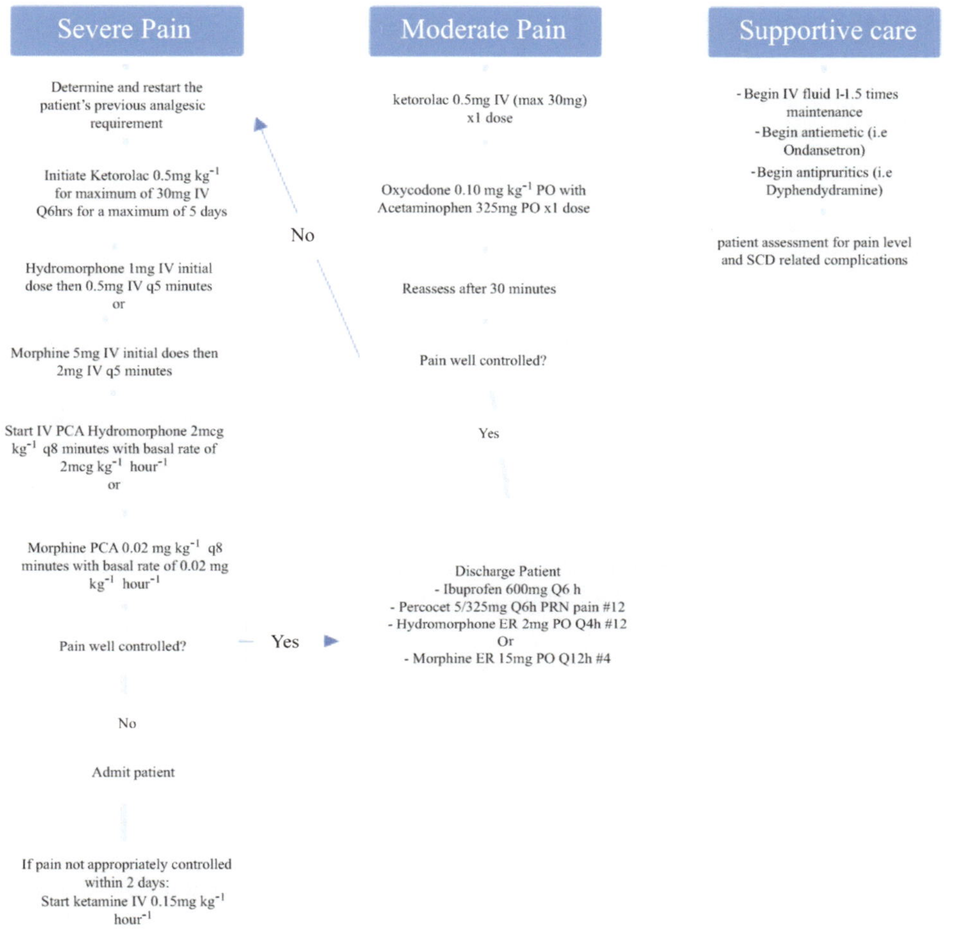

Figure 1. Management of SCD patient presenting to the ED with VOE.

This figure outlines our guidelines for the recommendation of the treatment of VOE in the ED.

Alternatively, institution that do not typically encounter individuals with SCD and that do not have an algorithm in place for the management of a patient that presents to their healthcare facility for the first time should involve starting with the lowest dose for the shortest duration possible in order to control the symptoms if the pain is mild to moderate and the patient has not been opioid naïve [39]. If the pain is moderate to severe and the patient has previously attempted an opioid medication without relief, a higher dose of opioid is preferred. From that baseline, the physician should titrate the dose, and duration of the analgesic medications upwards until adequate pain relief is achieved. On the other hand, as discussed earlier, the patient who presents for a subsequent visit to the same healthcare facility should initially be restarted on the same analgesic regimen with which adequate pain relief was obtained in the previous visits for VOE crises.

1.	Admission to the hospital
2.	Readmission to the hospital
3.	Length of stay in the ED or hospital
4.	Patient pain assessment (i.e., VAS, Baker-Wong faces scale)
5.	Patient satisfaction
6.	Parent satisfaction

Table 2. Indicators of effective/ineffective VOE treatment.

Whenever initiating opioid analgesia, it is mandatory to monitor for respiratory and sedation status. Useful questionnaires such as the Richmond Agitation Sedation Scale (RASS), the visual analogue scale (VAS) exist for sedation and pain assessment respectively. Respiratory status is typically monitored by pulse oximetry and visual assessment although some institution advocate for continuous end-tidal carbon dioxide monitoring ($EtCO_2$), especially when using high doses of opioids.

The preferred and recommended primary pharmacological method to treat the VOE crises is the opioid analgesic route and the commonly used medications include codeine, morphine, hydromorphone, fentanyl, hydrocodone/acetaminophen, hydrocodone/ibuprofen, oxymorphone, oxycodone, methadone and diamorphine [9].

3.2. Opioid medications

The first opiate used for VOE in the ED was meperidine in the 1960s. At home, short-acting oxycodone with acetaminophen was the most often used home medication. Morphine sulfate then got FDA approval in the 1980s and became the opiate of choice for the management of VOE in the 1990s. Not only did morphine show improvement in pain management and decreased hospital admissions related to VOE, it also did not possess the feared seizure side effect related to the meperidine metabolites, Normeperidine. These metabolites reduce the seizure threshold and also accumulate in patient with renal insufficiency, a complication commonly seen in patients with SCD [40–42]. In today's world though, as mentioned earlier, many different types of opioid are used effectively for the treatment of VOE-related pain but in the United States, intravenous hydromorphone is the drug most commonly used in the hospital setting and oral oxycodone as home prescription medications [43]. As a comparison, in the United Kingdom, intravenous morphine, diamorphine and oral oxycodone are the most commonly used pain medications for VOE pain.

Opioid agonists produce their effect by binding into μ receptors. The potency of a particular opioid is dependent on the binding affinity or strength with which that drug binds to its receptors and there is a great amount of variability of potency between different opiates. For example, hydromorphone is 5–7 as potent as morphine while sufentanyl is 500–1000 as potent as morphine. When an opiate binds to its receptors, it initiates a cascade of biochemical events that starts with activation of G-proteins, inhibition of adenylate cyclase activity and extrusion of K^{++} that result in hyperpolarisation of cell membranes, which delays or prevents the transmission of painful stimuli. Additionally, there exists a multitude of different receptors that each mediates the desired analgesic differently. Thus, the response to opioids depends not only on the type of opioid used, but also on the number and activity of the opioid receptors that a certain patient has. An opioid that binds a low number of receptors and has poor affinity, for example, is unlikely to produce effective analgesia in certain patients even if the dose is high. On the other hand, an opioid binding to an elevated number of receptors and with moderate or high binding affinity would provide effective analgesia even if used in small doses. This is part of the reason, among many others, why there is an immense variability to the pain response in patients with SCD. A dose considered an under treatment for a particular patient could overdose another patient.

3.3. Opioids adverse events

Unfortunately, opioids are not without side effects. The long list of mild to moderate adverse effects includes pruritus, nausea, vomiting, constipation, urinary retention, seizures, hives and the notorious respiratory depression. As mentioned earlier, seizures are mostly associated with meperidine. Other opioids have also possessed a potential for albeit a lot smaller and thought to be derived from the neuroexcitation related to metabolite of the opiate. Opioid-induced pruritus is one of the most prevalent complications with the use of opioids and is typically well controlled by either hydroxyzine, diphenhydramine, low dose naloxone and, now recognized as the most effective treatment, nalbuphine. The more serious complications, some of which are very popular topic of debates in the world today include addiction, tolerance, withdrawal, physical dependence and pseudoaddiction. A condition feared by many providers in today's world is addiction; a condition that is influenced by genetic, psychological and environmental factors that lead to compulsive use despite harm. Opiates are strong stimulants of the reward/pleasure system, increasing the level of dopamine in the system, which in turn enhances the desire to achieve the reward/pleasure. Addiction can ultimately lead to overdose and death. Tolerance, on the other hand, represents a state of adaptation in which exposure to the same amount of the drug results in a lower effect than previously obtained. Physical dependence also happens frequently and is the cause of the known withdrawal syndrome that manifests with abrupt cessation or an exaggerated reduction in the dose of opiate administered. Signs and symptoms of withdrawal include tremor, shakiness, anxiety, depression, lacrimation, rhinorrhea, fatigue, irritability, and diarrhea. Pseudoaddiction is very common in patients with SCD. It is a state, in which the patient appears to be seeking for excessive amount of medication, but is due to under-treatment of pain and resolves when the pain is treated properly. Opioid-induced hyperalgesia (OIH) results from chronic administration of opioid medications. A process that is not totally proven and well understood yet but is thought to result from a minor excitatory pathway that becomes magnified with chronic use of the opiates and, ultimately, becomes the dominant effect. The sites of pain from OIH are typically the same as the sites perceived during the VOE crisis, but the quality of the pain differs. It is more neuropathic in nature.

3.4. Nonsteroidal anti-inflammatory drugs

Nonsteroidal anti-inflammatory drugs (NSAIDs) are the main adjuvant of opioid in today's therapeutic guidelines of most healthcare facilities. Ketorolac tromethamine is the NSAID most commonly used for this purpose; it is commonly administered either intravenously or intramuscularly at a dose of 0.5 mg kg^{-1} for a maximum of 30 mg every 6 h for 5 days. NSAIDs partly inhibit the inflammatory cascade involved in VOE (see above). Although usually not sufficient to resolve a pain crisis as a sole treatment, it works synergistically with opioids. For moderate VOE pain, a single dose of 30 mg IV is typically sufficient. Opioids are limited by their propensity to cause gastritis and gastric bleeding. The drug should be used cautiously in patients with peptic ulcer disease or a history of gastrointestinal bleeding. NSAIDs can impair kidney function and accelerate the renal injury produced by sickle cell disease itself. For these reasons, many specialists avoid NSAIDs in patients with sickle cell disease.

3.5. Ketamine

Ketamine is gaining a lot of popularity for the treatment of VOE refractory to opioids. A lot of institutions have integrated its use in their algorithm of VOE treatment and strong evidence exists regarding its efficacy as an adjuvant to opioids and NSAIDs. Ketamine is a noncompetitive antagonist at the *N*-methyl-d-aspartate (NMDA) receptor. This property has been shown to modulate opioid tolerance and opioid-induced hyperalgesia. The use of ketamine is limited by its psychiatric side effects such as hallucinations, abnormal dreams, nightmares and abnormal behavior. Randomized controlled trials are still necessary for the regular implementation of ketamine in SCD protocols.

4. Pain management of patients with sickle cell disease with chronic and neuropathic pain

4.1. Chronic pain

In addition to the acute crises, patients with SCD also suffer from chronic pain, which often times overlap with acute pain crises and create difficulty in designing a treatment plan. These individuals can find management of their pain very difficult and therefore change providers frequently, resulting in a higher degree of misdiagnosis and misperception of their pain. Identifying the presenting syndrome can help individualize a treatment plan and therefore understanding the signs and symptoms of chronic pain is crucial for aggressive and effective therapy.

Chronic pain is generally defined as pain that is present for 3 or more months. As opposed to the acute pain, which is sharp and throbbing in nature with a sudden onset, chronic pain is often vague, deep, and achy there is present for a longer period. Approximately 5–10% of adult patients with sickle cell disease are affected with chronic pain [44]. However, a recent study from Pain in Sickle Cell Epidemiology Study reported the incidence of chronic pain in 29% of 292 adult patients [45]. These patients tend to be older and use more opioids [46]. The chronic pain is categorized into two types. The first type is objective and is due to visible signs such as leg ulcers and avascular necrosis which is associated with deep somatic pain. The second type is due to recurrent acute attacks of painful crises. Failure to treat these acute attacks can lead to chronic pain syndrome and resultant neuropathic pain. The exact pathophysiologic mechanism is not fully understood, however central component has been described in which the threshold for the perception of pain is lowered, resulting in pain from typically nonpainful stimuli (allodynia) and severe pain generated by mildly painful stimuli (hyperalgesia) (**Figure 2**).

This figure depicts the age distribution of SCD patient with chronic pain. As demonstrated by the figure, the larger proportion of SCD patients with chronic pain is between 20 and 29 years old.

4.2. Pathophysiology and mechanism

Although the exact mechanism underlying the transition from acute to chronic pain is not fully understood, some contributing factors include chronic inflammation, organ damage, and opioid-induced hyperalgesia [47]. According to a study presented at the Annual Meeting of American Society of Hematology, patients with chronic pain (defined as >50% of days reported as painful crises collected over 6 months) tend to be older (41 vs. 32 years), use more opioids (11.45 mg/day vs. 2.92 mg/day), and have higher levels of mast cell activation [48].

Opioid-induced hyperalgesia is a state of sensitization caused by repetitive exposure to opioids resulting in paradoxical response to pain. Although there is no understanding or consensus on the biomolecular mechanism, it is believed to be secondary to neuroplastic changes in the central and peripheral nervous system [49]. Despite it being a controversial topic, patients with sickle cell disease with chronic pain do require increasingly higher dosage adjustments.

Recent research demonstrates clear evidence that chronic inflammation and mast cell activation plays a role in the chronic pain state of patients with sickle cell disease. Mast cells release the neuropeptide substance P, which promotes neurogenic inflammation and nociceptive

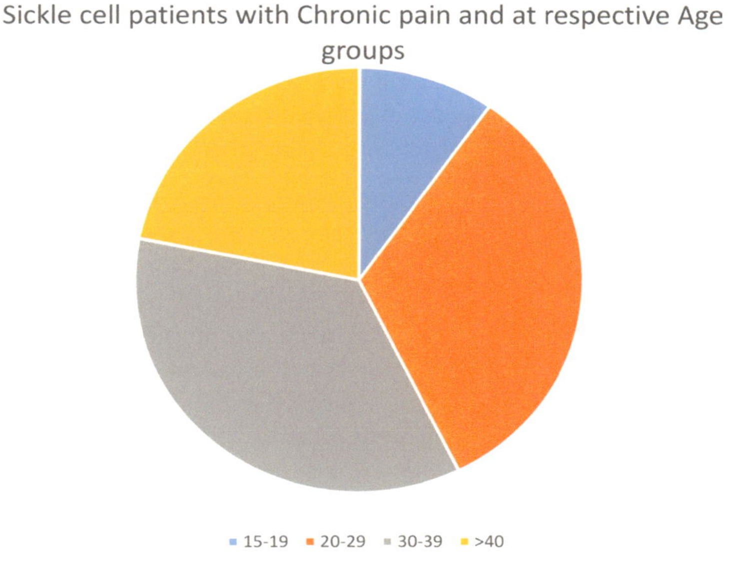

Figure 2. Distribution of SCD patient with chronic pain.

activation [48]. Additionally, tryptase, a serine proteinase found within mast cells appears far more elevated in patients with chronic pain in sickle cell disease. This can help guide future therapy directed toward inhibition of mast cell activation, and implementation of medications such as Cromolyn. This can also help identify and diagnose patients with sickle crises who present to the emergency department and are sadly mistaken as drug seeking opportunists.

4.3. Treatment/management

The cornerstone to therapy involves recognition of the disease state and assessment of the pain intensity, which helps individualize therapy. Prevention of SCD pain is crucial by avoidance of precipitating factors (dehydration, infection, diuretics, altitude, acidosis, and hypoxia), as repetitive acute inflammation can result in chronic pain. The approach to pain management in patients with SCD with chronic pain is multidisciplinary, involving the use of pharmacologic analgesic drugs, nerve blocks, physical therapy, and cognitive behavioral therapy [46]. Discussion of hydroxyurea and other disease modifying therapies is appropriate. Close attention should be made to psychosocial issues including depression and social isolation [45].

Mild chronic pain can be treated with acetaminophen or dihydrocodeine. In patients with liver failure, acetaminophen can be avoided and NSAIDS such as ibuprofen can be used, but should be used with caution in patients with borderline renal function or failure. In patients with moderate pain, consideration of slow release morphine with small amounts of rapid-release morphine for breakthrough pain is advised [46]. Alternatives to Morphine include hydromorphone, oxycodone, methadone, or transdermal fentanyl. Methadone in particular can be efficacious in patients with suspected opioid-induced hyperalgesia due to its N-methyl-D-aspartate (NMDA) antagonism and monoaminue uptake reuptake inhibition. In patients who cannot tolerate opioid side effects and have contraindications the prior listed opioid analgesics, tramadol, a selective Mu-receptor agonist and serotonin–norepinephrine reuptake inhibitor can be considered [44]. The goal of chronic pain management is to maximize the quality of life rather than short-term pain suppression [45]. Other adjuvants include partial opioid agonists such as buprenorphine, topical agents, corticosteroids, antihistamines, benzodiazepines, antidepressants, anticonvulsants, and phenothiazines.

In patients with severe chronic pain, alternative procedures can be considered in addition to opioid therapy. For example, in a patient with deep somatic pain of avascular necrosis of the hip, an interventional nerve block could supply instant relief for 12 h, and potentially 72 h if the injectate is liposomal Bupivacaine [49, 50]. Physiotherapy can help strengthen muscle fibers and loosen stiff joints, preventing contractures and physical disability. Psychological support with cognitive behavioral therapy can help the patient cope with pain or deal with the mental agony and psychosocial stressors associated with sickle cell disease [46]. Adapting to cognitive skills can also help alter the perception of pain as negative thinking has been linked to higher pain scores. Massage therapy, relaxation techniques, and even self-prayer have been reported in published studies to help with chronic pain [51]. The American Pain Society strongly recommends psychological, behavioral and physical modalities as necessary complements to pharmacologic therapy, as a significant effect on pain scores and activities of daily living have been reported [52]. Orthopedic devices for back or leg support can be deployed to reduce chronic pain in the hips or back. Orthopedic surgery, such as total hip replacement should be deferred until the pain is no longer tolerable [46].

Lastly, it important to note that patients with SCD are not immune to non-hemoglobinopathic pain. Excluding other disease processes is essential and misdiagnosis can be life threatening. Conditions that can mimic the chronic pain state include but are not limited to ischemic colitis, pancreatitis, bone marrow infarction, hepatobiliary disorders, and vertebral body necrosis [53].

4.4. Neuropathic pain

In addition to acute and chronic pain, a neuropathic component of pain plays a large and undiagnosed constituent of chronic disease. Data suggest that the development of neuropathic pain is responsible for the transition from acute to chronic pain with aging [54]. The general understanding is that multiple components of central sensitization and peripheral nerve injury are responsible. Types of neuropathic pain include peripheral neuropathic (caused by vaso-occlusive crises and neuropathies) and central neuropathic (caused by CNS damage, ictus, and central sensitization). Peripheral nerve injury and prostaglandin release can sensitize peripheral nerve endings and facilitate the transmission of pain along the A-delta and C fibers to the cerebral cortex [44]. The exact mechanism, however, is poorly understood, which hinders our progression toward achieving novel therapies.

Neuropathic pain from SCD occurs more commonly in older adults and females, which is hypothesized to be secondary to abnormalities in pain signaling pathways. These patients have extreme sensitivity to tactile touch (allodynia), increased pain from a normally painful stimulus (hyperalgesia) and extreme sensitivity to temperature [45]. Some studies demonstrate the prevalence to be approximately 20% of the chronic pain population. In a 2013 article published in Pediatric Blood and Cancer, 37% of patients with SCD were identified to have neuropathic pain and only 5% were reported to be taking a neuropathic pain drug (gabapentin), which highlights the lack of diagnosis and treatment [55]. Thus, appropriate screening tools such as the pain DETECT questionnaire could help identify patients with neuropathic pain and help initiate treatment.

4.5. Treatment/management

Although no single treatment therapy exists, a multimodal pharmacologic approach can be instituted in patients diagnosed with neuropathic pain. Treatment may include tricyclic antidepressants (TCA, SSRI, SNRIs, MAOIs) or anticonvulsants (pregabalin, gabapentin), although there is no data supporting its use in patients with SCD [56]. With a better safety profile and less side effects than opioids, tramadol (a typical analgesic with weak opioid receptor agonism and SNRI activity) can act centrally and be helpful in treating neuropathic pain, but should be used with caution in patients with renal failure [57, 58].

5. Future of SCD pain treatment

Until SCD can be fully cured (possibly with gene therapy), new and improved treatment modalities are necessary. The information currently available about SCD is that rapid and aggressive therapy at the first sign of a VOE help reduce the length of the event and even abort it. Currently, patients with VOE receive treatment 2–3 days after the onset of the prodromal signs [16]. Measurement should be made in the future to offer patients with SCD methods of treatment available at home such as opioids (IV or IM), supplemental oxygen, and rapid hydration methods. Anti-inflammatory agents and oral opioids represent the current home treatment modalities. Vasodilators also represent a fundamental therapeutic weapon for VOE, especially when used early. Administration of nitric oxide (NO) in the emergency department has shown to abort the crisis in some patients; however, no benefice was found when NO was used during the hospital stay [59–61]. Perhaps NO could be offer as a home medication and its use would be even earlier than it would be in the ED. Recently, reports have emerged of small doses of opioid antagonist in combination with an agonist enhanced the analgesic effect and delayed the development of tolerance [62]. Recent trials targeting the inhibition of the capsaicin receptor transient receptor potential vanillin 1 (TRPV1) showed promising results in relieving pain in patients with SCD [63].

6. Conclusion

Although many complications stem from SCD, leading to a significantly reduced lifespan, pain remains the most cardinal sign of the disease and is still inappropriately treated. The main explanations for the inadequate treatment are the providers' lack of knowledge about the disease and its narcotic requirement, lack of institutional treatment protocol in place and lack of patient education. The most important factors about the treatment, to our knowledge, are rapid and aggressive treatment as soon as signs of VOE happen, adequate rehydration and oxygenation. The treatment modalities have evolved enormously since the discovery of the disease and hopes for future treatment are bright.

Acknowledgements

To the entire staff of Advocate Illinois Masonic Medical Center, Dr. Arjang Khorasani, Dr. Kenneth Candido and Dr. Nick Knezevic, thank you for your continuous support throughout our work.

Author details

Thomas Zouki*, Armen Haroutunian and Tennison Malcolm

*Address all correspondence to: zoukit7@gmail.com

Department of Anesthesiology, Advocate Illinois Masonic Medical Center, Chicago, Illinois, USA

References

[1] Regional Committee for Africa 60. S-Cell Disease: A strategy for the WHO African Region. 2011 May 26 [cited 2018 Apr 28]. Available from: http://apps.who.int/iris/handle/10665/1682

[2] Bender MA. Sickle Cell Disease. In: Adam MP, Ardinger HH, Pagon RA, Wallace SE, Bean LJ, Stephens K, et al, editors. GeneReviews® [Internet]. Seattle (WA): University of Washington, Seattle; 1993 [cited 2018 Apr 28]. Available from: http://www.ncbi.nlm.nih.gov/books/NBK1377/

[3] Weatherall DJ, Clegg JB. Inherited haemoglobin disorders: An increasing global health problem. Bulletin of the World Health Organization. 2001;**79**(8):704-712

[4] CDC. Data and Statistics | Sickle Cell Disease | NCBDDD | CDC [Internet]. Centers for Disease Control and Prevention. 2016 [cited 2018 Apr 30]. Available from: https://www.cdc.gov/ncbddd/sicklecell/data.html

[5] Diallo D, Tchernia G. Sickle cell disease in Africa. Current Opinion in Hematology. 2002 Mar;**9**(2):111-116

[6] Scott RB. Health care priority and sickle cell anemia. JAMA [Internet]. 1970 Oct 26 [cited 2018 Apr 7];**214**(4):731-734. Available from: https://jamanetwork.com/journals/jama/fullarticle/357392

[7] Ballas SK. Update on pain management in sickle cell disease. Hemoglobin [Internet]. 2011 Oct 1 [cited 2018 Apr 5];**35**(5-6):520-529. Available from: https://doi.org/10.3109/03630269.2011.610478

[8] Frenette PS. Sickle cell vaso-occlusion: Multistep and multicellular paradigm. Current Opinion in Hematology. 2002 Mar;**9**(2):101-106

[9] Ballas SK. Current issues in sickle cell pain and its management. Hematology. American Society of Hematology. Education Program. 2007;**1**:97-105

[10] Plankton S, Haywood C, Segal JB, Dover GJ. Hospitalization rates and costs of care of patients with sickle-cell anaemia in the state of Maryland in the era of Hydroxyurea. American Journal of Haematology [Internet]. 2006 Dec 1 [cited 2018 Apr 4];**81**(12):927-932. Available from: https://onlinelibrary.wiley.com/doi/abs/10.1002/ajh.20703

[11] Ballas SK, Lusardi M. Hospital readmission for adult acute sickle cell painful episodes: frequency, etiology, and prognostic significance. American Journal of Hematology [Internet]. 2005 May 1 [cited 2018 May 23];**79**(1):17-25. Available from: https://onlinelibrary.wiley.com/doi/abs/10.1002/ajh.20336

[12] AlJuburi G, Laverty AA, Green SA, Phekoo KJ, Bell D, Majeed A. Socio-economic deprivation and risk of emergency readmission and inpatient mortality in people with sickle cell disease in England: observational study. Journal of Public Health (Oxford, England)

[Internet]. 2013 Dec 1 [cited 2018 May 23];**35**(4):510-517. Available from: https://academic.oup.com/jpubhealth/article/35/4/510/1686557

[13] Gill FM, Sleeper LA, Weiner SJ, et al. Clinical events in the first decade in a cohort of infants with sickle cell disease: Cooperative study of sickle cell diseae. Blood. 15 Jul 1995;**86**(2):776-783

[14] Powars DR. Natural history of sickle cell disease—The first ten years. Seminars in Hematology [Internet]. 1975 Jul 1 [cited 2018 May 23];**12**(3):267-285. Available from: https://www.seminhematol.org/article/0037-1963(75)90021-9/fulltext

[15] Jenkins TL. Sickle Cell Anemia in the Pediatric Intensive Care Unit: Novel Approaches for Managing Life-threatening Complications. AACN Advanced Critical Care [Internet]. 2002 May 1 [cited 2018 Apr 7];**13**(2):154-168. Available from: http://acc.aacnjournals.org/content/13/2/154

[16] Ballas SK, Gupta K, Adam-Graves P. Sickle cell pain: A critical reappraisal. Blood. August 2012;**120**(18):3647-3656

[17] Beyer JE, Simmons LE, Woods GM, Woods PM. A chronology of pain and comfort in children with sickle cell disease. Archives of Pediatrics & Adolescent Medicine [Internet]. 1999 Sep 1 [cited 2018 Apr 7];**153**(9):913-920. Available from: https://jamanetwork.com/journals/jamapediatrics/fullarticle/347703

[18] Jacob E, Beyer JE, Miaskowski C, Savedra M, Treadwell M, Styles L. Are there phases to the Vaso-occlusive painful episode in sickle cell disease? Journal of Pain and Symptom Management [Internet]. 2005 Apr 1 [cited 2018 Apr 7];**29**(4):392-400. Available from: http://www.jpsmjournal.com/article/S0885-3924(05)00050-3/abstract

[19] Ballas SK, Smith ED. Red blood cell changes during the evolution of the sickle cell painful crisis. Blood. 1992;**79**(8):2154-2163

[20] Jacob E, Mueller BU. Pain experience of children with sickle cell disease who had prolonged hospitalizations for acute painful episodes. Pain Medicine. 2008;**9**:13-21

[21] A Brief History of Sickle Cell Disease [Internet]. [cited 2018 Apr 30]. Available from: http://www.sicklecell.howard.edu/ABriefHistoryofSickleCellDisease.htm

[22] Diggs LW, Ching RE. Pathology of sickle cell anemia. Southern Medical Journal [Internet]. 1934 Oct 1 [cited 2018 Apr 30];**27**(10):839-845. Available from: https://insights.ovid.com/southern-medical/smeda/1934/10/000/pathology-sickle-cell-anemia/3/00007611

[23] Diggs LW, Williams DL. Treatment of Painful Sickle Cell Crises with Papaverine: Preliminary Report. Southern Medical Journal [Internet]. 1963 [cited 2018 Apr 30];**56**(5):472-474. Available from: https://www.cabdirect.org/cabdirect/abstract/19632901722

[24] Vichinsky EP, Neumayr LD, Earles AN, et al. Causes and outcomes of the acute chest syndrome in sickle cell disease. New England Journal of Medicine [Internet]. 2000 Jun 22 [cited 2018 May 23];**342**(25):1855-1865. Available from: https://doi.org/10.1056/NEJM200006223422502

[25] Hassell KL, Eckman JR, Lane PA. Acute multiorgan failure syndrome: A potentially catastrophic complication of severe sickle cell pain episodes. The American Journal of Medicine [Internet]. 1994 Feb 1 [cited 2018 May 23];**96**(2):155-162. Available from: http://www.sciencedirect.com/science/article/pii/0002934394901368

[26] Ngo S, Bartolucci P, Lobo D, Mekontso-Dessap A, et al. Causes of death in sickle cell disease adult patients: Old and new trends. Blood [Internet]. 2014 Dec 6 [cited 2018 May 23];**124**(21):2715. Available from: http://www.bloodjournal.org/content/124/21/2715

[27] De Ceulaer K, Gruber C, Hayes R, Serjeant GR. Medroxyprogesterone acetate and homozygous sickle-cell disease. Lancet. 1982 Jul 31;**2**(8292):229-231

[28] Ballas SK. Pain Management of Sickle Cell Disease. Hematology/Oncology Clinics of North America [Internet]. 2005 Oct [cited 2018 Apr 28];**19**(5):785-802. Available from: http://linkinghub.elsevier.com/retrieve/pii/S0889858805000894

[29] Gaston MH, Verter JI, Woods G, et al. Prophylaxis with oral penicillin in children with sickle cell anemia. A randomized trial. The New England Journal of Medicine. 1986 Jun 19;**314**(25):1593-1599

[30] Okomo U, Meremikwu MM. Fluid replacement therapy for acute episodes of pain in people with sickle cell disease. In: The Cochrane Library [Internet]. John Wiley & Sons, Ltd; 2017 [cited 2018 May 23]. Available from: http://cochranelibrary-wiley.com/doi/10.1002/14651858.CD005406.pub5/full

[31] Friedland LR, Pancioli AM, Duncan KM. Pediatric emergency department analgesic practice. Pediatric Emergency Care. 1997;**13**:103-106

[32] Brown DW. The dawn of healthy people 2020: A brief look back at its beginnings. Preventive Medicine. 2009;**48**:94-95

[33] Aisiku IP, Penberthy LT, Smith WR, et al. Patient satisfaction in specialized versus nonspecialized adult sickle cell care centers: The PiSCES study. Journal of the National Medical Association. 2007;**99**:886-890

[34] Ballas SK. Ethical issues in the management of sickle cell pain. American Journal of Hematology. 2001;**68**:127-132

[35] Jacob E, Miaskowski C, Savedra M, et al. Management of vaso-occlusive pain in children with sickle cell disease. Journal of Pediatric Hematology/Oncology. 2003;**25**:307-311

[36] Frenette PS, Atweh GF. Sickle cell disease: old discoveries, new concepts, and future promise [Internet]. 2007 [cited 2018 May 23]. Available from: https://www.jci.org/articles/view/30920/pdf

[37] Maxwell K, Streetly A, Bevan D. Experiences of hospital care and treatment-seeking behavior for pain from sickle cell disease: Qualitative study. The Western Journal of Medicine. 1999;**171**:306-313

[38] Rupp T, Delaney KA. Inadequate analgesia in emergency medicine. Annals of Emergency Medicine. 2004;**43**:494-503

[39] Sickle cell disease: Managing acute painful episodes in hospital. Guidance and guidelines. NICE [Internet]. [cited 2018 Apr 28]. Available from: https://www.nice.org.uk/guidance/cg143/chapter/1-recommendations

[40] Ballas SK, McCarthy WF, Guo N, et al. Early detection of response to Hydroxyurea therapy in patients with sickle cell Anemia. Hemoglobin [Internet]. 2010 Oct [cited 2018 Apr 29];**34**(5):424-429. Available from: https://www.ncbi.nlm.nih.gov/pubmed/20854115

[41] Ballas SK, Bauserman RL, McCarthy WF, et al. Utilization of analgesics in the multicenter study of hydroxyurea in sickle cell anemia: Effect of sex, age, and geographical location. American Journal of Hematology 2010 Aug;**85**(8):613-616

[42] Brookoff D, Polomano R. Treating sickle cell pain like Cancer pain. Annals of Internal Medicine. 1992 Apr 1;**116**:364-368

[43] Miller ST, Kim HY, Weiner D, et al. Inpatient management of sickle cell pain: A 'snapshot' of current practice. American Journal of Hematology. 2012;**87**:333-336

[44] Niscola P, Sorrentino F, Scaramucci L, De Fabritiis P, Cianciulli P. Pain syndromes in sickle cell disease: An update. Pain Medicine [Internet]. 2009 Apr 1 [cited 2018 May 1];**10**(3):470-480. Available from: https://academic.oup.com/painmedicine/article/10/3/470/1929112.

[45] Chen E, Cole SW, Kato PM. A review of empirically supported psychosocial interventions for pain and adherence outcomes in sickle cell disease. Journal of Pediatric Psychology. 2004 May;**29**(3):197-209

[46] Okpala I, Tawil A. Management of pain in sickle-cell disease. Journal of the Royal Society of Medicine [Internet]. 2002 Sep [cited 2018 May 1];**95**(9):456-458. Available from: https://www.ncbi.nlm.nih.gov/pmc/articles/PMC1279994/

[47] Pope M, Albo C, Kidwell KM, Xu H, Bowman L, Wells L, et al. Evolution of chronic pain in sickle cell disease. Blood [Internet]. 2016 Dec 2;**128**(22):1297. Available from: http://www.bloodjournal.org/content/128/22/1297.abstract

[48] Tennant F, MD, DrPH, Ciccone TG. New look at sickle cell patients with chronic pain [Internet]. Practical Pain Management. [cited 2018 May 1]. Available from: https://www.practicalpainmanagement.com/resources/news-and-research/new-look-sickle-cell-patients-chronic-pain

[49] Lee M, Silverman SM, Hansen H, Patel VB, Manchikanti L. A comprehensive review of opioid-induced hyperalgesia. Pain Physician. 2011 Apr;**14**(2):145-161

[50] Commissioner of the FDA. FDA In Brief: FDA approves new use of Exparel for nerve block pain relief following shoulder surgeries [Internet]. [cited 2018 May 1]. Available from: https://www.fda.gov/NewsEvents/Newsroom/FDAInBrief/ucm604021.htm

[51] Myers DC, Robinson EM, Guthrie HT, Lamp PS, Lottenberg R. Adjunctive approaches for sickle cell chronic pain. Complementary Health Practice Review. 1999 Dec 1;**5**:203-212

[52] Pain in Sickle-Cell Disease Guideline. APS [Internet]. [cited 2018 May 1]. Available from: http://americanpainsociety.org/education/guidelines/sickle-cell-guideline

[53] Al-Salem AH, Naserullah Z, Qaisaruddin S, Al-Abkari H, Al-Faraj A, Yassin YM. Splenic complications of the sickling syndromes and the role of splenectomy. J Pediatr Hematol Oncol [Internet]. 1999 [cited 2018 May 1];**21**(5):401-406. Available from: http://europepmc.org/abstract/med/10524454

[54] Fillingim RB. Individual differences in pain responses. Current Rheumatology Reports [Internet]. 2005 Sep 1 [cited 2018 May 23];**7**(5):342-347. Available from: https://link.springer.com/article/10.1007/s11926-005-0018-7

[55] Brandow AM, Farley RA, Panepinto JA. Neuropathic pain in patients with sickle cell disease. Pediatric Blood & Cancer. 2014 Mar;**61**(3):512-517

[56] Parikh RH. Patient-controlled analgesia improves pain control in a vaso-occlusive crisis in sickle cell patients. Clinical Research in Practice: The Journal of Team Hippocrates [Internet]. 2017 Sep 14 [cited 2018 May 1];**3**(2). Available from: http://digitalcommons.wayne.edu/crp/vol3/iss2/10

[57] Hollingshead J, Dühmke RM, Cornblath DR. Tramadol for neuropathic pain. Cochrane Database of Systematic Reviews. 2006 Jul 19;**3**:CD003726

[58] Stamer UM, Stüber F, Muders T, Musshoff F. Respiratory depression with tramadol in a patient with renal impairment and CYP2D6 gene duplication. Anesthesia & Analgesia [Internet]. 2008 Sep [cited 2018 May 23];**107**(3):926. Available from: https://journals.lww.com/anesthesia-analgesia/pages/articleviewer.aspx?year=2008&issue=09000&article=00035&type=Fulltext

[59] Gladwin MT, Kato GJ, Weiner D, Onyekwere OC, Dampier C, Hsu L, et al. Nitric oxide for inhalation in the acute treatment of sickle cell pain crisis: A randomized controlled trial. JAMA [Internet]. 2011 Mar 2 [cited 2018 Apr 30];**305**(9):893-902. Available from: https://jamanetwork.com/journals/jama/fullarticle/645928

[60] Lopez BL, Davis-Moon L, Ballas SK, Ma X. Sequential nitric oxide measurements during the emergency department treatment of acute vasoocclusive sickle cell crisis. American Journal of Hematology [Internet]. 2000 May 1 [cited 2018 May 23];**64**(1):15-19. Available from: https://onlinelibrary.wiley.com/doi/abs/10.1002/%28SICI%291096-8652%28200005%2964%3A1%3C15%3A%3AAID-AJH3%3E3.0.CO%3B2-P

[61] Head CA, Swerdlow P, McDade WA, et al. Beneficial effects of nitric oxide breathing in adult patients with sickle cell crisis. American Journal of Hematology [Internet]. 2010 Oct 1 [cited 2018 Apr 30];**85**(10):800-802. Available from: https://onlinelibrary.wiley.com/doi/abs/10.1002/ajh.21832

[62] Crain SM, Shen K-F. Antagonists of excitatory opioid receptor functions enhance morphine's analgesic potency and attenuate opioid tolerance/dependence liability: Pain [Internet]. 2000 Feb [cited 2018 Apr 30];**84**(2):121-131. Available from: http://content.wkhealth.com/linkback/openurl?sid=WKPTLP:landingpage&an=00006396-200002010-00002

[63] Hillery CA, Kerstein PC, Vilceanu D, et al. Transient receptor potential vanilloid 1 mediates pain in mice with severe sickle cell disease. Blood [Internet]. 2011 Sep 22 [cited 2018 Apr 30];**118**(12):3376-3383. Available from: http://www.bloodjournal.org/content/118/12/3376

Chapter 3

Is Chronic Post-Surgical Pain Preventable?

Abdulaziz Al-Mahrezi and Asma Al-Shidhani

Additional information is available at the end of the chapter

http://dx.doi.org/10.5772/intechopen.79500

Abstract

Chronic post-surgical pain (CPSP) is a common problem following surgery. It has significant impact on the patients' quality of life, chronic pain treatment services and resources in general. The prevalence of CPSP ranges between 5 and 50% of all surgical patients, but severe CPSP is present in less than 10% of the patients. The recognised potential risk factors for CPSP are young age, female gender, overweight, psychological factors, genetic tendency, pre-operative pain, surgery-related factors and severe post-operative pain. Hence, early identification of patients at risk will help to reduce the proportion of patients who are likely to develop CPSP. Different modalities of treatments or interventions are used to prevent the CPSP. These modalities include pre-emptive use of gabapentin, pregabalin or SNRIs, perioperative administration of ketamine, NSAIDs and steroids. In addition, the following interventions have been studied: surgical technique selection, regional and local anaesthesia, intrathecal administration of morphine and multimodal analgesia. Since the present evidence of these interventions is inconclusive because of methodological issues, further studies are still needed to develop more effective and evidence-based strategies to prevent CPSP.

Keywords: chronic pain, post-surgical pain, prevention, gabapentin, anaesthesia

1. Introduction

Millions of people undergo surgical interventions annually all over the world. A majority of them recover within a few days after surgery and go back to resume their routine daily activities. However, it is estimated that one out of five patients who undergo surgery do not completely recover and develop chronic post-surgical pain (CPSP) [1]. Indeed, surgery was identified as one of the most common causes for chronic pain among patients who attended pain clinics [2]. Although there is no universally accepted definition for CPSP, it is generally described as pain which persists after a surgical procedure beyond the surgical wound-healing time. There was no consensus about the time frame which defines chronicity following surgery, and this ranged from 1 month to 1 year [3]. However, more recently, an International Association for the Study of Pain (IASP) task force has defined the period as 3 months which is consistent with the definition of chronicity in other types of chronic pain [4]. In the quest for a clearer definition, Macrae proposed a four-point definition for CPSP. CPSP becomes chronic if (1) the pain has developed as a consequence of surgery, (2) its duration is at least 2 months, (3) no other explanation exists for the pain and (4) the pain is not a continuation of a pre-existing chronic pain condition for which the surgery was performed [5].

Studies have shown that the incidence of CPSP ranges from 5 to 50% [6]. Major surgical procedures such as mastectomy are associated with a higher incidence (20–50%), whereas minor procedures such as hernia repair are associated with a lower incidence (5–35%) [6]. Anatomically, the most affected sites are chest wall, breast, hip joints and iliac crest bone [1].

As any type of chronic pain, CPSP is considered as a major public health problem. It has a huge impact on the quality of life and psychological well-being. Chronic pain has been shown to affect mood, sleep and basic daily activities [7]. In severe cases, it can lead to disability. It is also associated with a heavy socio-economic burden as a result of direct costs which are related to treatment and indirect costs such as lost wages and unemployment [8]. Prevention is far more important than treatment here because of the incurable nature of CPSP and its association with neuropathic type of pain which is always difficult to treat.

Hence, the aim of this chapter is to review the pathophysiology of CPSP and to explore the risk factors which contribute to its development, bearing in mind the great importance of early identification of patients who are at risk before surgery. Different modalities of treatments and interventions, which have been used in the context of prevention of CPSP, will be discussed.

2. Pathophysiology

Understanding the pathophysiology of post-surgical pain is crucial for the development of effective approaches to prevent and treat the CPSP. Pain is a psychological sensory experience which is caused by different factors. These factors are nociceptive, inflammatory and neuropathic pain [9]. Two main mechanisms have been described to contribute towards the development of CPSP. These are inflammation and surgical injury to major peripheral nerves [6]. Tissue cutting and handling during any surgery causes the release of sensitising, inflammatory cell mediators. These mediators are cytokines, bradykinin and prostaglandins. These inflammatory mediators activate nociceptors which demonstrate reversible plasticity. Nociceptor stimuli are carried to the dorsal horn of the spinal cord via primary afferent Aδ and C fibres as electrical impulses. Moreover, those electrical impulses will be taken to the cerebral cortex and other higher centres via the contralateral spinothalamic and spinoreticular pathways: the two main ascending pain pathways which lead to the experience of pain. This process leads to the occurrence of peripheral and central sensitisation. The peripheral sensitisation enhances pain sensitivity at the site of tissue injury. It occurs when the activation threshold of nociceptors is lowered. This type of inflammatory pain, secondary to local excitability, usually subsides once the source of the mediators subsides, as tissue healing occurs or the disease process is controlled. Non-steroidal anti-inflammatory drugs (NSAIDs) inhibit the production of prostaglandin E2 via locally induced cyclooxygenase-2 enzymes and hence reduce peripheral sensitisation and pain. By contrast, the central sensitisation is an excitability of neurons in the central nervous system (CNS). It occurs because of enhanced pain signalling within the spinal cord in the second-order neurons due to ongoing nociceptive input which may last longer than the initial stimulus. Clinically, this manifests as wind-up, long-term potentiation, hyperalgesia and pain secondary to normally non-painful tactile stimuli (allodynia). Wind-up happens with the repeated activation of C fibres. Under normal conditions, due to the action of glutamate at N-methyl-D-aspartate (NMDA) receptors, a magnesium ion blocks the NMDA receptor. However, due to the presence of continuous painful stimuli, the response of second-order neurons to painful stimuli is amplified due to the removal of the magnesium block. This explains the role of ketamine (NMDA receptor antagonist) in reducing

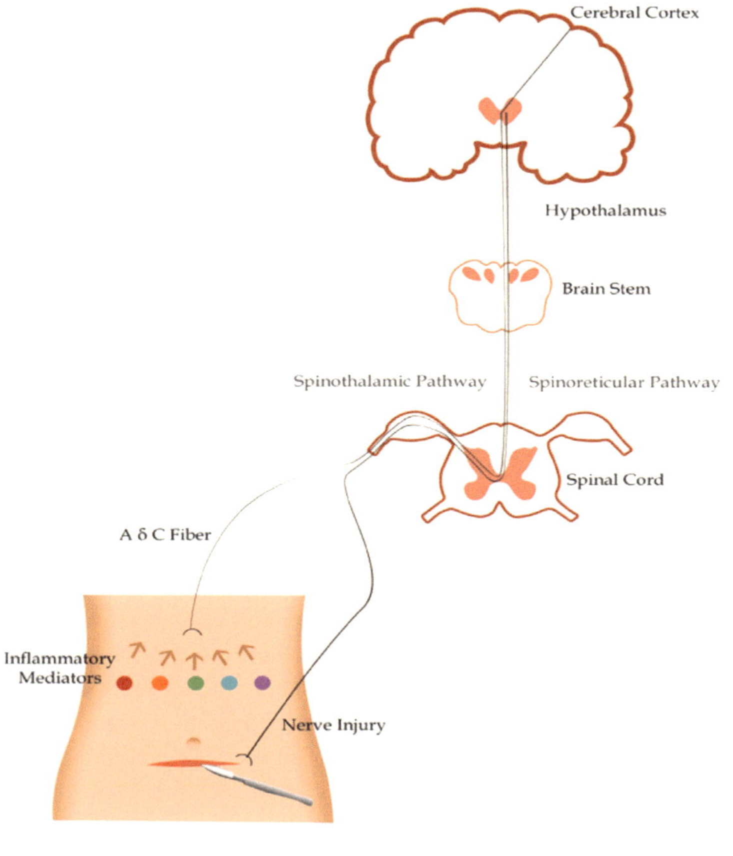

Figure 1. An illustration of the two main mechanisms which contribute towards the development of CPSP (inflammation and nerve damage). The pain pathways depicted here are the ascending pain pathways [10].

or blocking wind-up. The long-term potentiation is the second-order neurons response which last longer than the initial stimulus. Hyperalgesia results from an amplified response to painful stimuli due to both long-term potentiation and lowering of the pain threshold outside of the area of inflammation [10].

Nerve damage is the second major contributor for the development of CPSP. It is very important here to try to explore the mechanisms of differentiation of neuropathic from non-neuropathic pain. In most affected patients, the pain component of CPSP is similar to pain experienced as a result of neuropathic pain [11, 12]. In patients with CPSP, neuropathic pain can occur as a consequence of spontaneous ectopic discharges from damaged nerves and nearby undamaged nerves following nerve injury. Furthermore, disinhibition of pain pathways and facilitation of pain transmission occur due to loss of inhibitory interneurons in the dorsal horn. Hypoesthesia and neuropathic pain are both caused by nerve damage. In addition, the presence of hypoesthesia in CPSP patients confirms the association between nerve damage and CPSP [11, 12]. Thoracotomy is a good example of surgeries which may lead to nerve injury. In thoracotomy, the use of a rib retractor blocks intercostal nerve conduction by 50–100% in segments close to the incision [13]. Moreover, the degree of nerve damage in thoracotomy correlates with the intensity of chronic pain [14]. In conclusion, acute and chronic pain experience is a multifactorial complex process, involving physiological, genetic and psychosocial factors. These factors contribute to the conversion of somatosensory activity into a pain experience, to the amplitude of and reaction to the sensation, and to related changes in mood and behaviour [9] (**Figure 1**).

3. Risk factors

Various risk factors have been postulated to predict the development of chronic post-surgical pain in patients undergoing surgical procedures [9]. These factors are; genetic susceptibility, preceding pain, acute post-operative pain, psychosocial factors, demographic factors and surgical factors. These factors can be classified as patient-related and medical factors or to modifiable and non-modifiable risk factors [6, 10]. Each factor will be discussed separately in the subsequent text (**Figure 2**).

3.1. Genetic susceptibility

Different people respond differently to physiological and clinical pain because of the variation in pain sensitivity. This discrepancy in pain sensitivity is a recognised factor for susceptibility to CPSP and response to analgesia [15–19]. There are strong indications that chronic pain and specifically CPSP are heritable traits and that genetic variation accounts for about half of the difference in pain levels. Studies done on rodents pointed to a strong heritable component of susceptibility to develop neuropathic pain, but the responsible genes have not yet been identified [19–21]. Future exploration of pain genetic may lead towards a remarkable improvement in CPSP treatment and to a more specific and personalised pain medicine [22]. Analysis of patients' DNA sequences of pain biomarkers and their analgesic responses to

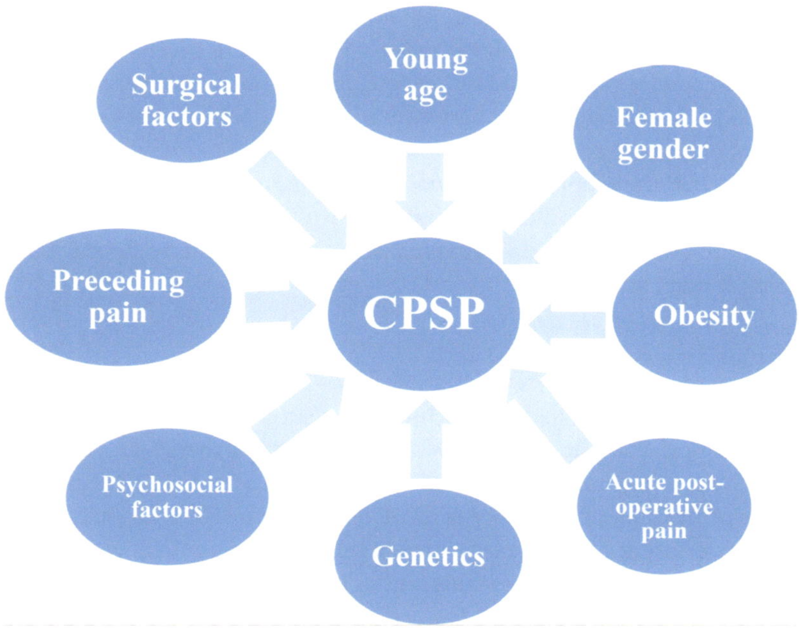

Figure 2. Potential risk factors for CPSP development.

medications will facilitate better understanding of CPSP pathophysiology, and thus it will help to predict a patient's likelihood of developing CPSP even before surgery. In addition, these advances could help in providing effective treatment regimens that will prevent the transition to chronic pain post surgically and help to provide treatment for those who had already developed CPSP. The genetic role is further highlighted by the experimental studies which were done on catecholamine-O-methyltransferase (COMT). In these studies, a correlation was found between the increased COMT activities and the risk of developing chronic temporo-mandibular joint pain [17, 18]. Many investigators have proposed that some clinical disorders such as fibromyalgia, migraine, irritable bowel syndrome, irritable bladder and Raynaud's syndrome could be considered as markers of post-injury chronic pain [23, 24]. In view of the complexity of neuropathic pain, it is very likely that more than one single gene might contribute to the development of CPSP [9].

3.2. Preceding pain and acute post-operative pain

Multiple studies looked at the effect of perioperative pain on the development of chronic post-surgical pain [25–34]. The factors mainly studied were the level of pain immediately before the surgery, the presence of previous chronic pain (lasting more than 6 months) before the surgery and acute pain at post-operative period. The first two factors have independently predicted moderate to intense pain in the acute post-operative period [25, 26]. Three studies, which were done on patients who underwent hernia repair and amputation surgeries, reported that the presence of pre-operative pain at the site of the operation or closer to it can predict chronic pain after the surgery [30, 33, 34]. In addition, the patients who experienced more severe and long lasting pain before the surgery felt more severe pain after the surgery compared to patients who experienced less severe pain before the surgery [29, 30]. Finally, the last factor studied was the correlation between immediate post-operative pain intensity and the development of chronic post-operative pain [31, 32]. Studies found an increase of two- to threefold risk of CPSP development in patients with immediate post-operative pain [34]. In conclusion, these associations indicate the potential for the prevention of CPSP by aggressive control of pain both pre- and post-operatively and by addressing any chronic pain issues well before planning for any surgery.

3.3. Demographic factors

Younger patients are more likely to develop chronic postsurgical pain than older patients [35–40]. Smith et al. [35] found that chronic pain was seen in 65% of the 30–49 years' age group, in 40% of the 50–69 years' age group, and in 26% of patients older than 70 years. Another study showed that the probability of incidence of CPSP decreased by 5% with each 1 year increase in age in women undergoing breast cancer surgery [41]. Similar findings were seen after hernia repair surgery [36]. The explanation for this higher incidence of CPSP in younger age group is not yet known, but it might be related to the reduction in peripheral nociceptive function with increased age [9]. Besides age, gender has also been identified as another demographic factor. Studies showed that women have higher post-operative pain than men [42, 43]. Furthermore, angina patients with a higher body mass index (BMI ≥ 25) pre-operatively or at the time of surgery were more likely to report CPSP [40]. A young obese female has been described as the triad of high risk to develop CPSP in any patient undergoing surgery [6, 9, 42].

3.4. Psychosocial factors

Previous studies focused on biological factors as predictors for the development of CPSP, but recently, the evidence moved more towards a biopsychosocial model. Multiple pre-operative psychological factors have been studied. These are as follows: negative affective constructs such as anxiety symptoms, depressive symptoms, pain catastrophising, general psychological distress, perceived injustice and sensitivity to pain traumatization [44–57]. Patients with state-trait anxiety are believed to be more hypersensitive and psychologically more reactive to threatening stimuli [44, 57]. Studies showed that pre-operative anxiety and depression are correlated with a higher post-operative anxiety, a higher post-operative pain intensity, higher analgesia requirements and a longer length of hospital stay [44]. Fear of surgery was associated with more pain, poor recovery and a poor quality of life 6 months post-operatively. In one study done on patients who underwent breast cancer surgery, emotional distress like anxiety, depression, illness behaviour and somato-sensory amplification were reported as significant risk factors for higher post-operative acute pain at 1 month, but were not significantly correlated to persistent pain at 3 months post-operatively [58, 59]. On the other hand, a large prospective study with a sample size of 625 patients who had undergone minor, intermediate and major operative procedures found that the fear of the long-term consequences of surgery had predicted an increased level of pain at 6 months post-operatively [60]. This finding was independent of the type of surgical procedure and other somatic factors. In addition, research has explored the role of health-related beliefs, including catastrophising, in predicting CPSP. Catastrophising, claimed to be a trait-like characteristic, had mainly been assessed in non-surgical chronic pain populations or within the acute post-operative period [61, 62]. Studies reported that pre-operative catastrophising was the strongest independent predictor of pain ratings 2 years after knee arthroplasty [51, 63]. Also, patients who presented with pre-surgical anxiety and pre-surgical pain catastrophising before surgery were approximately twice as likely to develop CPSP compared with controls [64]. Furthermore, perceived injustice and sensitivity to pain traumatization might predict CPSP, but only a few studies were done and further research is still needed [52, 55, 56]. On the other hand, high dispositional optimism, high positive affect, low emotional distress, expectation of pain control and expectations about functional recovery before surgery were significantly associated with a lower pain intensity and fewer physical symptoms following surgery and a lower incidence of CPSP at 4 months in women undergoing breast cancer surgery. Taken altogether, these studies indicate that fostering optimism and enhancing self-efficacy and adaptive behaviours in the perioperative period may help patients navigate through their post-surgical recovery period [58, 65]. However, facing an uncertain future with the presence of health problems, and the requirement from the patient to bear significant pain and functional impairment of important daily activities during the recovery stage from major surgery makes it difficult for patients to always maintain an optimistic attitude [66]. Nevertheless, one study found that lower pre-operative pain self-efficacy scores, which assess a person's confidence in performing general activities despite pain, to be a significant predictor of greater functional limitations, but not pain, at 1 year after total knee arthroplasty [67]. While another study also done in patients undergoing total knee arthroplasty has shown that patients with a higher pre-surgical score on the Patient Activation Measure (reflecting the propensity to engage in adaptive health behaviours) experienced better pain relief at 6 months [68]. In conclusion, fear of surgery was the most consistent psychological predictor of unfavourable outcome, whereas dispositional optimism was related to a better long-term functional recovery after surgery. Further studies are still needed to develop a better understanding of the interaction between CPSP and psychosocial factors.

3.5. Surgical factors

Multiple surgical factors are related to the development of CPSP. These factors are the duration of the operation, surgical technique (laparoscopy vs. open), incision site and type, the experience of the surgeon and the centre where the intervention is performed [6]. In one study, researchers found that patients who underwent operations lasting more than 3 h had more chronic pain, poor functional outcome and poor global recovery at 6 months post-operatively [60]. Generally, the more serious the medical problem or more complicated, the more complex and longer the surgery [6]. Operations with a longer duration are associated with more surgical trauma, more persistent surgical nociception and sustained peripheral injury which in turn would trigger pathological changes in the central nervous system (CNS) [6, 9, 69, 70]. There is a strong relationship between the technique of surgery and the incidence of CPSP. Evidence showed that the more severe the surgical insult or tissue damage, the greater the risk of persistent pain. Significant differences were seen between open and laparoscopic procedures with a higher incidence of CPSP after open surgeries [71–73]. These findings were observed in different types of surgeries (hernia repair, cholecystectomy and hysterectomy) [71–73]. Less tissue handling and less intervention result in a lower incidence of chronic pain development. Wallace et al. [74] reported that the incidence of CPSP varied from 53% for mastectomy with reconstruction by implant, to 31% for mastectomy only, to 22% for breast reduction. Also, nerve protection during cutting and tissue handling in the operation site or in the neighbourhood during the perioperative period may decrease the incidence of CPSP. This is explained by the fact that nerve injury produces acute and lasting changes not only in the damaged nerves but also in the adjacent intact nerves [75]. Such effects would activate the pain pathways in the CNS, and motor and sympathetic systems [75]. The experience of the surgical team and the centre where the intervention took place have an impact on both morbidity and mortality [76]. CPSP was observed more commonly in surgical units with a lower number of cases and limited experience [76].

4. Potential for prevention

All surgeries carry the risk of CPSP but not all surgeries are medically necessary to be done. Clinicians are looking to moderate the risks of CPSP by identifying patients who are at a high risk prior to the surgical procedure. The identification of high-risk patients can be used to a closer monitoring of these patients and to initiate timely interventions to prevent chronic pain. Assessment tools can be used before surgery to identify the risk probability of developing CPSP by including some predictors such as age, sex, pre-operative pain, type of surgery, incision size, and level of anxiety, among others [77]. Several modalities and interventions have been investigated in the context of prevention of CPSP. Each of these modalities will be discussed in the following parts of this chapter.

4.1. Pre-emptive and preventive analgesia

Pre-emptive analgesia is delivered prior to skin incision. It is initiated before the surgical procedure in order to reduce peripheral and central pain pathways sensitization.

4.1.1. Gabapentin

Gabapentin has a well-established role in the treatment of several neuropathic pain conditions. It is also known to possess anti-nociceptive effects. Such effects result partially from its high affinity for the α 2 d subunit on pre-synaptic voltage-gated calcium channels, which are often upregulated following nerve injury. This leads to the inhibition of calcium influx and to the release of excitatory neurotransmitters, which produce central sensitization and the sensation of pain [78]. The use of gabapentin in CPSP has been extensively studied. The recent evidence indicated that perioperative gabapentin was effective in preventing CPSP. One recent meta-analysis supported the view that the perioperative administration of gabapentin was effective in reducing the incidence of CPSP [79]. Clarke et al. concluded that out of eight studies, four found that the perioperative administration of gabapentin decreased the incidence of chronic pain more than 2 months after surgery. Six out of the eight studies measured pain 6 months after surgery, and the pooled results demonstrated a moderate to large reduction in the development of CPSP (pooled odds ratio (OR) 0.52; 95% confidence interval (CI), 0.27–0.98; P 0.04) [79]. Two other studies, which investigated the effect of administering 1200 mg of gabapentin before surgery with placebo, reported a reduction in the incidence and severity of CPSP 6 months post -surgery [80, 81]. On the other hand, a systematic review done by Chaparro et al. [82] indicated that the effect of gabapentin was equivalent to placebo in preventing CPSP. Variations were observed in these studies in both the doses of gabapentin which were used (ranged from 300 to 1200 mg per day) and the duration of use (1 h before surgery to 10 days post surgery) [82]. Other variables, which could account for the conflicting evidence for the effectiveness of gabapentin, include diverse surgical procedures and small sample size.

4.1.2. Pregabalin

Pregabalin is a structural analogue of c-aminobutyric acid. It binds to the α 2 δ subunit of the voltage-gated calcium channel which subsequently lead to a decrease in the release of neurotransmitters such as glutamate, norepinephrine and substance P, thereby targeting the putative role of these transmitters in central sensitization in a similar way to gabapentin [83]. Chaparro et al. [82] conducted a systematic review in which five pregabalin trials with long-term pain outcomes were included. Two different dosing regimens were used in these clinical trials, either 150 mg 2 h prior to the induction of anaesthesia and 75 mg twice daily for two post-operative days or a 300-mg single dose pre-operatively followed by a 14-day twice-a-day (BID =50–150 mg). The heterogeneity (I2 of 28.5%) of dosing regimens was problematic with respect to comparing long-term outcomes. Two studies demonstrated a significant benefit of pregabalin as compared to placebo [84, 85]. While the pain outcomes differed at 3 months follow-up, an overall significant effect of pregabalin was reported [82]. Moreover, two additional studies showed a significant reduction in the incidence of CPSP 6 months following both total knee arthroplasty and off-pump coronary artery bypass surgery [84–86]. Therefore, despite the heterogeneity between studies, the available literature favours the perioperative use of pregabalin to prevent CPSP; however, the use of a high dose of pregabalin (300 mg) has been associated with serious adverse effects such as visual disturbances, sedation and confusion during the first day after surgery [85, 87, 88]. These adverse effects settled with continued use, but led to an overall recommendation of using lower doses of pregabalin, with the aim of reducing side effects and hence allowing the successful introduction of physiotherapy and intensive rehabilitation during the immediate post-operative period [85, 87, 88].

4.1.3. Selective norepinephrine and serotonin re-uptake inhibitors (SNRIs)

Venlafaxine hydrochloride is a selective norepinephrine and serotonin re-uptake inhibitor which is widely used as an antidepressant medication. It has a good safety profile as it does not bind to cholinergic, histamine or alpha 1-adrenergic receptors . The efficacy of Venlafaxine, which was administered perioperatively in patients with acute and chronic postmastectomy pain, has been investigated. The study concluded that venlafaxine significantly reduced the incidence of CPSP at 6 months . Duloxetine is another SNRI medication which has been effectively used in chronic neuropathic pain in patients with diabetic peripheral neuropathy and fibromyalgia [89–93]. However, its role in the prevention of CPSP has not been studied. The current evidence regarding the use of SNRIs in the prevention of CPSP is insufficient, and further studies are still needed.

4.2. Perioperative prevention

4.2.1. Surgical technique

Since nerve damage is considered as one of the major causes of chronic postsurgical pain, minimising nerve injury during any surgery is crucial. Nerve damage can be prevented or minimised by adopting several surgical techniques such as laparoscopic surgery, precise dissection during open surgery, the use of a lightweight mesh for inguinal hernia repair and the use of an intracostal suturing technique. Studies showed that laparoscopic herniorrhaphy and minimally invasive thoracoscopic techniques might decrease the risk of nerve damage and pain when compared with open surgery [94–96]. In addition, the avoidance of nerve damage by making more precise dissection during open surgery or by using the intracostal suturing technique to avoid direct nerve compression was also suggested to reduce the occurrence of CPSP [13, 97]. The use of a lightweight mesh in inguinal hernia repair was intended to produce less inflammatory response which would result in a reduction in the risk of CPSP [98, 99].

4.2.2. Regional anaesthesia

Regional anaesthesia is defined as the use of local anaesthetics to block the conduction of impulses along nerves and to minimise the transmission of signals to or within the spinal cord. Possibly, they prevent central sensitisation by preventing the nociceptive inputs into the dorsal horn [10]. Examples of regional anaesthesia are spinal and epidural techniques which act on the nerve roots. A recent Cochrane review concluded that epidural analgesia and paravertebral blocks were effective in reducing the risk of CPSP at 6 months after thoracotomy and breast cancer surgery, respectively [100], whereas a study by Capdevila et al. [101] did not show any benefit for epidural analgesia in reducing CPSP intensity after open nephrectomy. Spinal anaesthesia has also been shown to be beneficial compared to general anaesthesia in reducing the risk of chronic pain after caesarean section [102]. When comparing the route of regional anaesthesia, similar outcomes for paravertebral block (PVB) and thoracic epidural analgesia (TEA) were achieved [103]. In addition, a comparison between either of these techniques and opioids alone favoured RA [104]. Evidence was in favour for PVB for breast surgery and TEA for lung surgery [105]. The findings of these studies cannot be generalised to other surgical procedures due to small sample size and the experience of the centre where the procedure was conducted. In addition, the studies were heterogeneous in terms of agents used and routes of delivery. Currently, the available evidence suggests that regional anaesthetics as a class are equivocal to placebo for CPSP.

4.2.3. Intravenous lidocaine

Lidocaine is a local anaesthetic which possesses analgesic, anti-hyperalgesic and anti-inflammatory properties. It is usually given intravenously, and it is used as part of a multimodal analgesic regimen. Five studies found significant effects on the incidence of CPSP following the administration of perioperative intravenous lidocaine infusion in several types of surgeries (breast surgery, robot-assisted thyroidectomy and nephrectomy) at 6 months post surgery [106–110]. In conclusion, the available literature supports the use of intravenous lidocaine to prevent CPSP after specific surgical procedures.

4.2.4. Ketamine

Ketamine is a non-competitive NMDA receptor antagonist. The NMDA receptor plays a critical role in both the induction and maintenance of central sensitization and pathological pain. Ketamine is thought to reduce pain and analgesia consumption by preventing NMDA-mediated sensitization of the dorsal horn neurons in the spinal cord [111]. Generally, the available evidence supports the perioperative use of ketamine to prevent CPSP. The effects of ketamine on CPSP were investigated in 14 clinical trials, out of which, 12 trials were of good quality to be included in a systematic review [82]. In most of these trials, pre-incisional loading doses of ketamine, which ranged from 0.15 to 1 mg kg^{-1}, plus an intraoperative infusion was administered. While ketamine was not better than placebo for the reduction of CPSP at 3 months after surgery, a subgroup analysis of trials which only included patients who received ketamine for longer than 24 h demonstrated ketamine's superiority over placebo. A more definitive result was found for ketamine at 6 months following surgery, with an overall significant decrease in the incidence of CPSP. Interestingly, at 6 months following surgery, studies in which patients had received ketamine for less than 24 h demonstrated a reduction in the incidence of CPSP compared to studies in which ketamine was given for more than 24 h. The two clinical trials which were excluded from the systematic review reported no significant differences between ketamine and placebo [81, 112]. The reason for their exclusion was due to lack of reporting of the outcomes of interest. While the use of ketamine to reduce CPSP is empirically promising, the results still remain controversial due to the wide variability in clinical settings, ketamine dose and duration, and reported outcomes. In addition, some of the positive results were obtained using clinical anaesthesia regimens which are not accepted as standard treatments [112, 113]. Overall, the available literature supports the perioperative use of ketamine to prevent CPSP.

4.2.5. Intrathecal administration of morphine

Moriyama et al. [114] studied the effect of intrathecal administration of 0.1 mg morphine in women undergoing caesarean section during surgery. No respiratory depression was reported. The study concluded that although no effect on acute pain was observed, intrathecal administration of morphine significantly decreased chronic pain after surgery by 50% at 3 months post-operatively [114].

4.2.6. Multimodal analgesia

Multimodal analgesia has become the widely accepted modality of treatment for perioperative pain. It is utilising different regimens of different classes of medications according to the type of the surgical procedure and the institute where surgery is performed [115]. The main aim of multimodal analgesia is to target several peripheral and CNS mechanisms to maximise pain reduction, reduce opioids requirements and to decrease opioid-related side effects [103, 107]. A few studies have explored the effects of multimodal analgesia on CPSP prevention. The evidence indicated positive effects at 3 months [116] and at 1 year following surgery [117]. Additional studies are required to study the effects of multimodal analgesia on different types of surgical procedures and to find out whether its preventive effects do indeed reduce the incidence and severity of CPSP.

4.2.7. Non-steroidal anti-inflammatory drugs (NSAIDs)

Prostaglandins are one of the inflammatory mediators activated during surgery which has a possible role in CPSP pathophysiology. NSAIDs are a group of medications which are widely used for their anti-inflammatory properties. They reduce the pain and inflammation through the inhibition of the synthesis of prostaglandins by inhibiting COX-1 and COX-2 receptors. NSAIDs can reduce secondary hyperalgesia and central sensitization [118, 119]. One study showed that Celecoxib (COX-2 inhibitor) had reduced post-operative pain, the need for post-operative opioid analgesia [120] and meanwhile did not inhibit bone healing following arthroplasty surgery [121]. In summary, the available clinical trials are heterogeneous and differ in the following: the type of drug used, follow-up time point and pain outcomes. None of these trials demonstrated a significant impact of NSAIDs on reduction in the incidence or severity of CPSP [122, 123].

4.2.8. Glucocorticoids

Glucocorticoids prevent pain by expressing anti-inflammatory properties and by preventing central sensitization [124]. Three trials studied the effects of perioperative corticosteroid on CPSP. The studies used different types of steroids Dexamethasone, Methylprednisolone and Hydrocortisone. A Cochrane review included these clinical trials. The results were inconclusive, and the heterogeneity precluded any possible meta-analysis. The heterogeneity was due to variations in drugs used, follow-up time intervals and the measured pain outcomes [82].

5. Future directions

CPSP remains as a challenging clinical problem. There are several areas which are promising and can be explored further in the future. Investigators could focus more on the better

http://dx.doi.org/10.5772/intechopen.79500

identification of individual risk factors and the development of assessment tools before planning for any surgical procedure. There is a hope that we can develop better understanding about the genetics of pain to try to identify responsible genes and develop specific therapies for them. Future studies could be designed to be more procedure-specific to help us understand the mechanistic differences between surgical incisions and pathologies. The role of the multimodal analgesia in the prevention of CPSP should be explored further in view of the positive results of the few available studies. Advance in surgical techniques to try to minimise nerve injuries as much as possible since nerve damage plays a major role in the development of chronic postsurgical neuropathic pain is another promising area for research. Future studies in the field of CPSP should be designed in a better way to include a larger sample size, standard doses and regimens of drugs, and more consistent outcome measurement tools.

6. Conclusion

CPSP is a complex process which is not fully understood. When it occurs, it affects the patients' quality of life. Based on our current understanding of the pathophysiology, nerve injury and inflammation are the two main responsible mechanisms for the development of CPSP. Specific risk factors, which make some individuals at a higher risk than others for CPSP, have been identified. Timely identification of these individuals based on their risk profile allows us to develop appropriate interventions. Several modalities and interventions for CPSP prevention have been investigated. These include pre-emptive and perioperative interventions (**Table 1**). CPSP prevention is an important area for future research in view of the methodological problems with the majority of available studies.

1. Screen preoperatively for psychological problems such as anxiety, depression, and stress, and identify those patients for special attention, especially if they are having a high-risk procedure
2. Control preoperative pain aggressively.
3. Consider the perioperative use of gabapentin or pregabalin or ketamine.
4. Use epidural analgesia for thoracotomy and major laparotomy and paravertebral blockade for breast surgery.
5. If regional anaesthesia is not practical, consider perioperative intravenous lidocaine infusion.
6. Control immediate postoperative pain aggressively and for as long as necessary by any appropriate means.

Adapted with permission from reference [125].

Table 1. Evidence-based strategies to reduce the risk of chronic post-surgical pain (CPSP).

Author details

Abdulaziz Al-Mahrezi* and Asma Al-Shidhani

*Address all correspondence to: abdulaziz@squ.edu.om

Department of Family Medicine and Public Health, College of Medicine and Health Sciences, Sultan Qaboos University, Muscat, Oman

References

[1] Haroutiunian S, Nikolajsen L, Finnerup NB, Jensen TS. The neuropathic component in persistent postsurgical pain: A systematic literature review. Pain. 2013;**154**:95-102. DOI: 10.1016/j.pain.2012.09.010

[2] Crombie IK, Davies HTO, Macrae WA. Cut and thrust: Antecedent surgery and trauma among patients attending a chronic pain clinic. Pain. 1998;**76**:167-171. DOI: 10.1016/S0304-3959(98)00038-4

[3] Reichling DB, Levine JD. Critical role of nociceptor plasticity in chronic pain. Trends in Neurosciences. 2009;**32**:611-618. DOI: 10.1016/j.tins.2009.07.007

[4] Treede RD, Rief W, Barke A, et al. A classification of chronic pain for ICD-11. Pain. 2015;**156**:1003-1007. DOI: 10.1097/j.pain.0000000000000160

[5] Macrae WA. Chronic post-surgical pain: 10 years on. British Journal of Anaesthesia. 2008;**101**:77-86. DOI: 10.1093/bja/aen099

[6] Akkaya T, Ozkan D. Chronic post-surgical pain. Agrı. 2009;**21**(1):1-9

[7] Raftery MN, Sarma K, Murphy AW, De la Harpe D, Normand C, McGuire BE. Chronic pain in the Republic of Ireland--community prevalence, psychosocial profile and predictors of pain-related disability: Results from the prevalence, impact and cost of chronic pain (PRIME) study, part 1. Pain. 2011;**152**:1096-1103. DOI: 10.1016/j.pain.2011.01.019

[8] Leadley RM, Armstrong N, Lee YC, Allen A, Kleijnen J. Chronic diseases in the European Union: The prevalence and health cost implications of chronic pain. Journal of Pain and Palliative Care Pharmacotherapy. 2012;**26**:310-325. DOI: 10.3109/15360288.2012.736933

[9] Kehlet H, Troels SJ, Clifford JW. Persistent postsurgical pain: Risk factors and prevention. Lancet. 2006;**367**:1618-1625. DOI: 10.1016/S0140-6736(06)68700-X

[10] Reddi D, Curran N. Chronic pain after surgery: Pathophysiology, risk factors and prevention. Postgraduate Medical Journal. 2014;**90**:222-227. DOI: 10.1136/postgradmedj-2013-132215

[11] Mikkelsen T, Werner MU, Lassen B, Kehlet H. Pain and sensory dysfunction 6 to 12 months after inguinal herniotomy. Anesthesia and Analgesia. 2004;**99**:146-151. DOI: 10.1213/01.ANE.0000115147.14626.C5

[12] Jung BF, Ahrendt GM, Oaklander AL, Dworkin RH. Neuropathic pain following breast cancer surgery: Proposed classification and research update. Pain. 2003;**104**: 1-13. DOI: 10.1016/S0304-3959(03)00241-0

[13] Rogers ML, Henderson L, Mahajan RP, Duffy JP. Preliminary findings in the neurophysiological assessment of intercostal nerve injury during thoracotomy. European Journal of Cardio-Thoracic Surgery. 2002;**21**:298-301. DOI: 10.1016/S1010-7940(01)01104-6

[14] Benedetti F, Vighetti S, Ricco C, Amanzio M. Neurophysiologic assessment of nerve impairment in posterolateral and muscle-sparing thoracotomy. The Journal of Thoracic and Cardiovascular Surgery. 1998;**115**:841-847. DOI: 10.1016/S0022-5223(98)70365-4

[15] Hartvigsen J, Christensen K, Frederiksen H, Pedersen HC. Genetic and environmental contributions to back pain in old age: A study of 2,108 Danish twins aged 70 and older. Spine. 2004;**29**:897-901

[16] Hakim AJ, Cherkas L, El Zayat S, MacGregor AJ, Spector TD. The genetic contribution to carpal tunnel syndrome in women: A twin study. Arthritis and Rheumatism. 2002;**47**:275-279. DOI: 10.1002/art.10395

[17] Zubieta JK, Heitzeg MM, Smith YR, et al. COMT val158met genotype affects mu-opioid neurotransmitter responses to a pain stressor. Science. 2003;**299**:1240-1243. DOI: 10.1126/science.1078546

[18] Diatchenko L, Slade GD, Nackley AG, et al. Genetic basis for individual variations in pain perception and the development of a chronic pain condition. Human Molecular Genetics. 2005;**14**:135-143. DOI: 10.1093/hmg/ddi013

[19] Mogil JS, Wilson SG, Chesler EJ, et al. The melanocortin-1 receptor gene mediates female-specific mechanisms of analgesia in mice and humans. Proceedings of the National Academy of Sciences of the United States of America. 2003;**100**:4867-4872. DOI: 10.1073/pnas.0730053100

[20] Mogil JS, Yu L, Basbaum AI. Pain genes? Natural variation and transgenic mutants. Annual Review of Neuroscience. 2000;**23**:777-811. DOI: 10.1146/annurev.neuro.23.1.777

[21] Devor M, Raber P. Heritability of symptoms in an experimental model of neuropathic pain. Pain. 1990;**42**:51-67. DOI: 10.1016/0304-3959(90)91092-W

[22] Clarke H, Katz J, Flor H, Rietschel M, Seltzer SRZ. Genetics of chronic post-surgical pain: A crucial step toward personal pain medicine. Canadian Journal of Anesthesia. 2015;**62**:294-303. DOI: 10.1007/s12630-014-0287-6

[23] Courtney CA, Duffy K, Serpell MG, O'Dwyer PJ. Outcome of patients with severe chronic pain following repair of groin hernia. The British Journal of Surgery. 2002;**89**:1310-1314. DOI: 10.1046/j.1365-2168.2002.02206.x

[24] Wright D, Paterson C, Scott N, Hair A, O'Dwyer PJ. Five-year follow-up of patients undergoing laparoscopic or open groin hernia repair: A randomized controlled trial. Annals of Surgery. 2002;**235**:333-337

[25] Bhave G, Gereau RW. Posttranslational mechanisms of peripheral sensitization. Journal of Neurobiology. 2004;**61**:88-106. DOI: 10.1002/neu.20083

[26] Julius D, Basbaum AI. Molecular mechanisms of nociception. Nature. 2001;**413**:203-210. DOI: 10.1038/35093019

[27] Ji RR, Kohno T, Moore KA, Woolf CJ. Central sensitization and LTP: Do pain and memory share similar mechanisms. Trends in Neurosciences. 2003;**26**:696-705. DOI: 10.1016/j.tins.2003.09.017

[28] Samad TA, Moore KA, Sapirstein A. al. Interleukin-1betamediated induction of COX-2 in the CNS contributes to inflammatory pain hypersensitivity. Nature. 2001;**410**:471-475. DOI: 10.1038/35068566

[29] Jensen TS, Krebs B, Nielsen J, Rasmussen P. Immediate and long term phantom limb pain in amputees: Incidence, clinical characteristics and relationship to pre-amputation limb pain. Pain. 1985;**21**:267-278. DOI: 10.1016/0304-3959(85)90090-9

[30] Nikolajsen L, Ilkjaer S, Kroner K, Christensen JH, Jensen TS. The influence of preamputation pain on postamputation stump and phantom pain. Pain. 1997;**72**:393-405

[31] Tasmuth T, Estlanderb AM, Kalso E. Effect of present pain and mood on the memory of past postoperative pain in women treated surgically for breast cancer. Pain. 1996;**68**:343-347. DOI: 10.1016/S0304-3959(96)03219-8

[32] Katz J, Jackson M, Kavanagh BP, Sandler AN. Acute pain after thoracic surgery predicts long-term post-thoracotomy pain. The Clinical Journal of Pain. 1996;**12**:50-55

[33] Callesen T, Bech K, Kehlet H. Prospective study of chronic pain after groin hernia repair. The British Journal of Surgery. 1999;**86**:1528-1531. DOI: 10.1046/j.1365-2168.1999.01320.x

[34] Poobalan AS, Bruce J, Smith WC, King PM, Krukowski ZH, Chambers WA. A review of chronic pain after inguinal herniorrhaphy. The Clinical Journal of Pain. 2003;**19**:48-54

[35] Smith WCS, Bourne D, Squair J, Phillips DO, Chambers WA. A retrospective cohort study of post mastectomy pain syndrome. Pain. 1999;**83**:91-95

[36] Poobalan AS, Bruce J, King PM, Chambers WA, Krukowski ZH, Smith WC. Chronic pain and quality of life following open inguinal hernia repair. The British Journal of Surgery. 2001;**88**:1122-1126. DOI: 10.1046/j.0007-1323.2001.01828.x

[37] Andersen KG, Kehlet H. Persistent pain after breast cancer treatment: A critical review of risk factors and strategies for prevention. The Journal of Pain. 2011;**12**:725-746. DOI: 10.1016/j.jpain.2010.12.005

[38] Wildgaard K, Ravn J, Nikolajsen L, Jakobsen E, Jensen TS, Kehlet H. Consequences of persistent pain after lung cancer surgery: A nationwide questionnaire study. Acta Anaesthesiologica Scandinavica. 2011;**55**:60-68. DOI: 10.1111/j.1399-6576.2010.02357.x

[39] Gjeilo KH, Klepstad P, Wahba A, Lydersen S, Stenseth R. Chronic pain after cardiac surgery: A prospective study. Acta Anaesthesiologica Scandinavica. 2010;**54**:70-78. DOI: 10.1111/j.1399-6576.2009.02097.x

[40] Bruce J, Drury N, Poobalan AS, Jeffrey RR, Smith WC, Chambers WA. The prevalence of chronic chest and leg pain following cardiac surgery: A historical cohort study. Pain. 2003;**104**:265-273

[41] Poleshuck EL, Katz J, Andrus CH, et al. Risk factors for chronic pain following breast cancer surgery: A prospective study. The Journal of Pain. 2006;**7**:626-634. DOI: 10.1016/j.jpain.2006.02.007

[42] Katz J, Poleshuck EL, Andrus CH, et al. Risk factors for acute pain and its persistence following breast cancer surgery. Pain. 2005;**119**:16-25. DOI: 10.1016/j.pain.2005.09.008

[43] Gjeilo KH, Stenseth R, Klepstad P. Risk factors and early pharmacological interventions to prevent chronic postsurgical pain following cardiac surgery. American Journal of Cardiovascular Drugs. 2014;**14**:335-342. DOI: 10.1007/s40256-014-0083-2

[44] Caumo W, Schmidt AP, Schneider CN, et al. Preoperative predictors of moderate to intense acute postoperative pain in patients undergoing abdominal surgery. Acta Anaesthesiologica Scandinavica 2002;**46**:1265-1271. DOI.org/10.1034/j.1399-6576.2002.461015.x

[45] Masselin-Dubois A, Attal N, Fletcher D, et al. Are psychological predictors of chronic postsurgical pain dependent on the surgical model? A comparison of total knee arthroplasty and breast surgery for cancer. The Journal of Pain. 2013;**14**:854-864. DOI: 10.1016/j.jpain.2013.02.013

[46] Pinto PR, McIntyre T, Nogueira-Silva C, Almeida A, Araújo-Soares V. Risk factors for persistent postsurgical pain in women undergoing hysterectomy due to benign causes: A prospective predictive study. The Journal of Pain. 2012;**13**:1045-1057. DOI: 10.1016/j.jpain.2012.07.014

[47] Singh JA, Lewallen DG. Medical and psychological comorbidity predicts poor pain outcomes after total knee arthroplasty. Rheumatology. 2013;**52**:916-923. DOI: 10.1093/rheumatology/kes402

[48] Papakostidou I, Dailiana ZH. Papapolychroniou T, al. Factors affecting the quality of life after total knee arthroplasties: A prospective study. BMC Musculoskel Dis. 2012;**13**:116. DOI: 10.1186/1471-2474-13-116

[49] Sinikallio S, Airaksinen O, Aalto T, Lehto SM, Kröger H, Viinamäki H. Coexistence of pain and depression predicts poor 2-year surgery outcome among lumbar spinal stenosis patients. Nordic Journal of Psychiatry. 2010;**64**:391-396. DOI: 10.3109/08039481003759193

[50] Sinikallio S, Lehto SM, Aalto T, Airaksinen O, Kröger H, Viinamäki H. Depressive symptoms during rehabilitation period predict poor outcome of lumbar spinal stenosis surgery: A two-year perspective. BMC Musculoskeletal Disorders. 2010;**11**:152. DOI: 10.1186/1471-2474-11-152

[51] Riddle DL, Wade JB, Jiranek WA, Kong X. Preoperative pain catastrophizing predicts pain outcome after knee arthroplasty. Clinical Orthopaedics and Related Research. 2010;**468**:798-806. DOI: 10.1007/s11999-009-0963-y

[52] Yakobov E, Scott W, Stanish W, Dunbar M, Richardson G, Sullivan M. The role of perceived injustice in the prediction of pain and function after total knee arthroplasty. Pain. 2014;**155**:2040-2046. DOI: 10.1016/j.pain.2014.07.007

[53] Lingard EA, Riddle DL. Impact of psychological distress on pain and function following knee arthroplasty. The Journal of Bone and Joint Surgery. American Volume. 2007;**89**:1161-1169. DOI: 10.2106/JBJS.F.00914

[54] Mejdahl MK, Mertz BG, Bidstrup PE, Andersen KG. Preoperative distress predicts persistent pain after breast cancer treatment: A prospective cohort study. Journal of the National Comprehensive Cancer Network. 2015;**13**:995-1003. DOI: 10.6004/jnccn.2015.0120

[55] Kleiman V, Clarke H, Katz J. Sensitivity to pain traumatization: A higher-order factor underlying painrelated anxiety, pain catastrophizing and anxiety sensitivity among patients scheduled for major surgery. Pain Research and Management. 2011;**16**:169-177

[56] Katz J, Fashler SR, Wicks C, et al. Sensitivity to pain traumatization scale: Development, validation, and preliminary findings. Journal of Pain Research. 2017;**10**:1297-1316. DOI: 10.2147/JPR.S134133

[57] Johnston M, Vöegle C. Benefits of psychological preparation for surgery: A meta-analysis. Annals of Behavioral Medicine. 1993;**15**(4):245-256

[58] Ronaldson A, Poole L, Kidd T, Leigh E, Jahangiri M, Steptoe A. Optimism measured pre-operatively is associated with reduced pain intensity and physical symptom reporting after coronary artery bypass graft surgery. Journal of Psychosomatic Research. 2014;**77**:278-282. DOI: 10.1016/j.jpsychores.2014.07.018

[59] Langer E, Janis I, Wolfer J. Reduction of psychological stress in surgical patients. Journal of Experimental Social Psychology. 1975;**11**:115-165

[60] Peters ML, Sommer M, de Rijke JM, et al. Somatic and psychologic predictors of long-term unfavourable outcome after surgical intervention. Annals of Surgery 2007;245: 487-494. DOI: 10.1097/01.sla.0000245495.79781.65

[61] Sullivan MJL, Bishop SR, Pivik J. The pain catastrophizing scale: Development and validation. Psychological Assessment. 1995;**7**:524-532. DOI: 10.1037//1040-3590.7.4.524

[62] Granot M, Ferber SG. The roles of catastrophising and anxiety in the prediction of postoperative pain intensity: A prospective study. The Clinical Journal of Pain. 2005;**21**: 439-445. DOI: 10.1097/01.ajp.0000135236.12705.2d

[63] Forsythe ME, Dunbar MJ, Hennigar AW, Sullivan MJ, Gross M. Prospective relation between catastrophising and residual pain following knee arthoplasty: Two-year follow-up. Pain Research and Management. 2008;**13**(4):335-341

[64] Theunissen M, Peters ML, Bruce J, Gramke HF, Marcus MA. Preoperative anxiety and catastrophizing: A systematic review and meta-analysis of the association with chronic postsurgical pain. The Clinical Journal of Pain. 2012;**28**:819-841. DOI: 10.1097/AJP.0b013e31824549d6

[65] Bruce J, Thornton AJ, Powell R, et al. Psychological surgical, and sociodemographic predictors of pain outcomes after breast cancer surgery: A population-based cohort study. Pain. 2014;**155**:232-243. DOI: 10.1016/j.pain.2013.09.028

[66] Weinrib AZ, Azam MA, Birnie KA, Burns LC, Clarke H, Katz J. The psychology of chronic post-surgical pain: New frontiers in risk factor identification, prevention and management. British Journal of Pain. 2017;**11**:169-177. DOI: 10.1177/2049463717720636

[67] Wylde V, Dixon S, Blom A. The role of preoperative self-efficacy in predicting outcome after total knee replacement. Musculoskeletal Care. 2012;**10**:110-118. DOI: 10.1002/msc.1008

[68] Andrawis J, Akhavan S, Chan V, Lehil M, Pong D, Bozic KJ. Higher preoperative patient activation associated with better patient reported outcomes after total joint arthroplasty. Clinical Orthopaedics and Related Research. 2015;**473**:2688-2697. DOI: 10.1007/s11999-015-4247-4

[69] Bruce J, Quinlan J. Chronic post surgical pain. Reviews in Pain. 2011;**5**:23-29. DOI: 10.1177/204946371100500306

[70] Lavand'homme P, Thienpont E. Pain after total knee arthroplasty: A narrative review focusing on the stratification of patients at risk for persistent pain. Bone and Joint Journal. 2015;**97-B**(10 Suppl A):45-48. DOI: 10.1302/0301-620X.97B10.36524

[71] Callesen T, Kehlet H. Postherniorrhaphy pain. Anesthesiology. 1997;**87**:1219-1230

[72] Stiff G, Rhodes M, Kelly A, Telford K, Armstrong CP, Rees BI. Long-term pain: Less common after laparoscopic than open cholecystectomy. The British Journal of Surgery. 1994;**81**:1368-1370. DOI: 10.1002/bjs.1800810939

[73] Brandsborg B, Nikolajsen L, Hansen CT, Kehlet H, Jensen TS. Risk factors for chronic pain after hysterectomy: A nationwide questionnaire and database study. Anesthesiology. 2007;**106**:1003-1012. DOI: 10.1097/01.anes.0000265161.39932.e8

[74] Wallace MS, Wallace AM, Lee J, Dobke MK. Pain after breast surgery: A survey of 282 women. Pain. 1996;**66**:195-205. DOI: 10.1016/0304-3959(96)03064-3

[75] Devor M, Seltzer Z. Pathophysiology of damaged nerves in relation to chronic pain. In: Wall PD, Melzack R, editors. Textbook of Pain. Edinburgh, UK: Churchill Livingstone; 1999. pp. 129-164

[76] Tasmuth T, Blomqvist C, Kalso E. Chronic post-treatment symptoms in patients with breast cancer operated in different surgical units. European Journal of Surgical Oncology. 1999;**25**:38-43. DOI: 10.1053/ejso.1998.0597

[77] Janssen KJ, Kalkman CJ, Grobbee DE, Bonsel GJ, Moons KG, Vergouwe Y. The risk of severe postoperative pain: Modification and validation of a clinical prediction rule. Anesthesia and Analgesia. 2008;**107**:1330-1339. DOI: 10.1213/ane.0b013e31818227da

[78] Luo ZD, Calcutt NA, Higuera ES, et al. Injury type-specific calcium channel alpha 2 delta-1 subunit up-regulation in rat neuropathic pain models correlates with antiallodynic

effects of gabapentin. The Journal of Pharmacology and Experimental Therapeutics. 2002;**303**:1199-1205. DOI: 10.1124/jpet.102.041574

[79] Clarke H, Bonin RP, Orser BA, Englesakis M, Wijeysundera DN, Katz J. The prevention of chronic postsurgical pain using gabapentin and pregabalin. Anesthesia and Analgesia. 2012;**115**:428-442. DOI: 10.1213/ANE.0b013e318249d36e

[80] Sen H, Sizlan A, Yanarates O, et al. A comparison of gabapentin and ketamine in acute and chronic pain after hysterectomy. Anesthesia and Analgesia. 2009;**109**:1645-1650. DOI: 10.1213/ANE.0b013e3181b65ea0

[81] Sen H, Sizlan A, Yanarates O, et al. The effects of gabapentin on acute and chronic pain after inguinal herniorrhaphy. European Journal of Anaesthesiology. 2009;**26**:772-776. DOI: 10.1097/EJA.0b013e32832ad2fa

[82] Chaparro LE, Smith SA, Moore RA, Wiffen PJ, Gilron I. Pharmacotherapy for the prevention of chronic pain after surgery in adults. Cochrane Database of Systematic Reviews. 2013;**7**:CD008307. DOI: 10.1002/14651858.CD008307.pub2

[83] Herrero JF, Laird JM, Lopez-Garcia JA. Wind-up of spinal cord neurones and pain sensation: Much ado about something? Progress in Neurobiology. 2000;**61**:169-203. DOI: 10.1016/S0301-0082(99)00051-9

[84] Pesonen A, Suojaranta-Ylinen R, Hammaren E, et al. Pregabalin has an opioid-sparing effect in elderly patients after cardiac surgery: A randomized placebo-controlled trial. British Journal of Anaesthesia. 2011;**106**:873-881. DOI: 10.1093/bja/aer083

[85] Buvanendran A, Kroin JS, Della Valle CJ, Kari M, Moric M, Tuman KJ. Perioperative oral pregabalin reduces chronic pain after total knee arthroplasty: A prospective, randomized, controlled trial. Anesthesia and Analgesia. 2010;**110**:199-207. DOI: 10.1213/ANE.0b013e3181c4273a

[86] Joshi SS, Jagadeesh AM. Efficacy of perioperative pregabalin in acute and chronic post-operative pain after off-pump coronary artery bypass surgery: A randomized, double-blind placebo controlled trial. Annals of Cardiac Anaesthesia. 2013;**16**:180-185. DOI: 10.4103/0971-9784.114239

[87] Burke SM, Shorten GD. Perioperative pregabalin improves pain and functional outcomes 3 months after lumbar discectomy. Anesthesia and Analgesia. 2010;**110**:1180-1185. DOI: 10.1213/ANE.0b013e3181cf949a

[88] Anwar S, O'Brien B. The role of intraoperative interventions to minimize chronic post-surgical pain. British Journal of Pain. 2017;**11**:186-191. DOI: 10.1177/2049463717720640

[89] Taylor K, Rowbotham MC. Venlafaxine hydrochloride and chronic pain. The Western Journal of Medicine. 1996;**165**:147-148

[90] Amr YM, Yousef AA. Evaluation of efficacy of the perioperative administration of venlafaxine or gabapentin on acute and chronic postmastectomy pain. The Clinical Journal of Pain. 2010;**26**:381-385. DOI: 10.1097/AJP.0b013e3181cb406e

[91] Yasuda H, Hotta N, Nakao K, Kasuga M, Kashiwagi A, Kawamori R. Superiority of duloxetine to placebo in improving diabetic neuropathic pain: Results of a randomized controlled trial in Japan. The Journal of Diabetes Investigation. 2011;**2**:132-139. DOI: 10.1111/j.2040-1124.2010.00073.x

[92] Raskin J, Pritchett YL, Wang F, et al. A double-blind, randomized multicenter trial comparing duloxetine with placebo in the management of diabetic peripheral neuropathic pain. Pain Medicine. 2005;**6**:346-356. DOI: 10.1111/j.1526-4637.2005.00061.x

[93] Wernicke JF, Pritchett YL, D'Souza DN, et al. A randomized controlled trial of duloxetine in diabetic peripheral neuropathic pain. Neurology. 2006;**67**(8):1411-1420. DOI: 10.1212/01.wnl.0000240225.04000.1a

[94] Aasvang E, Kehlet H. Chronic postoperative pain: The case of inguinal herniorrhaphy. British Journal of Anaesthesia. 2005;**95**:69-76. DOI: 10.1093/bja/aei019

[95] Grant AM, Scott NW, O'Dwyer PJ. MRC. Laparoscopic groin hernia trial group. Five-year follow-up of a randomized trial to assess pain and numbness after laparoscopic or open repair of groin hernia. The British Journal of Surgery. 2004;**91**:1570-1574. DOI: 10.1002/bjs.4799

[96] Perkins FM, Kehlet H. Chronic pain as an outcome of surgery: A review of predictive factors. Anesthesiology. 2000;**93**:1123-1133

[97] Cerfolio RJ, Price TN, Bryant AS, Bass CS, Bartolucci AA. Intracostal sutures decrease the pain of thoracotomy. The Annals of Thoracic Surgery. 2003;**76**:407-412. DOI: 10.1016/S0003-4975(03)00447-8

[98] Picchio M, Palimento D, Attanasio U, Matarazzo PF, Bambini C, Caliendo A. Randomised controlled trial of preservation or elective division of ilioinguinal nerve on open inguinal hernia repair with polypropylene mesh. Archives of Surgery. 2004;**139**:755-758. DOI: 10.1001/archsurg.139.7.755

[99] O'Dwyer PJ, Kingsnorth AN, Molloy RG, Small PK, Lammers B, Horeyseck G. Randomised clinical trial assessing impact of a lightweight or heavyweight mesh on chronic pain after inguinal hernia repair. The British Journal of Surgery. 2005;**92**:166-170. DOI: 10.1002/bjs.4833

[100] Andreae MH, Andreae DA. Local anaesthetics and regional anaesthesia for preventing chronic pain after surgery. Cochrane Database of Systematic Reviews. 2012;(10)

[101] Capdevila X, Moulard S, Plasse C, Peshaud J-L, Molinari N, Dadure C, et al. Effectiveness of epidural analgesia, continuous surgical site analgesia, and patient-controlled analgesic morphine for postoperative pain management and hyperalgesia, rehabilitation, and health-related quality of life after open nephrectomy. Anesthesia and Analgesia. 2017;**124**:336-345

[102] Nikolajsen L, Sørensen HC, Jensen TS, et al. Chronic pain following caesarean section. Acta Anaesthesiologica Scandinavica. 2004;**48**:111-116

[103] Powell ES, Cook D, Pearce AC, et al. A prospective, multicentre, observational cohort study of analgesia and outcome after pneumonectomy. British Journal of Anaesthesia. 2011;**106**(3):364-370

[104] Senturk M, Ozcan PE, Talu GK, et al. The effects of three different analgesia techniques on long-term postthoracotomy pain. Anesthesia and Analgesia. 2002;**94**(1):11-15

[105] Andreae MH, Andreae DA. Regional anaesthesia to prevent chronic pain after surgery: A Cochrane systematic review and meta-analysis. British Journal of Anaesthesia. 2013;**111**(5):711-720

[106] Grigoras A, Lee P, Sattar F, Shorten G. Perioperative intravenous lidocaine decreases the incidence of persistent pain after breast surgery. The Clinical Journal of Pain. 2012;**28**:567-572. DOI: 10.1097/AJP.0b013e31823b9cc8

[107] Terkawi AS, Sharma S, Durieux ME, Thammishetti S, Brenin D, Tiouririne M. Perioperative lidocaine infusion reduces the incidence of post-mastectomy chronic pain: A double-blind, placebo-controlled randomized trial. Pain Physician. 2015;**18**:E139

[108] Kim MH, Lee K-Y, Park S, Kim SI, Park HS, Yoo YC. Effects of systemic lidocaine versus magnesium administration on postoperative functional recovery and chronic pain in patients undergoing breast cancer surgery: A prospective, randomized, double-blind, comparative clinical trial. PLoS One. 2017;**12**:e0173026-e0173013

[109] Choi KW, Nam KH, Lee JR, Chung WY, Kang SW, Joe YE, et al. The effects of intravenous lidocaine infusions on the quality of recovery and chronic pain after robotic thyroidectomy: A randomized, double-blinded controlled study. World Journal of Surgery. 2017;**41**:1305-1312

[110] Jendoubi A, Naceur I, Bouzouita A, Trifa M, Ghedira S, Chebil M, et al. A comparison between intravenous lidocaine and ketamine on acute and chronic pain after open nephrectomy: A prospective, double-blind, randomized, placebo-controlled study. Saudi Journal of Anaesthesia. 2017;**11**:177

[111] Woolf CJ, Chong MS. Preemptive analgesia–treating postoperative pain by preventing the establishment of central sensitization. Anesthesia and Analgesia. 1993;**77**:362-379

[112] Dullenkopf A, Muller R, Dillmann F, Wiedemeier P, Hegi TR, Gautschi S. An intraoperative pre-incision single dose of intravenous ketamine does not have an effect on postoperative, analgesic requirements under clinical conditions. Anaesthesia and Intensive Care. 2009;**37**:753-757

[113] Elia N, Tramer MR. Ketamine and postoperative pain: A quantitative systematic review of randomised trials. Pain. 2005;**113**:61-70. DOI: 10.1016/j.pain.2004.09.036

[114] Moriyama K, Ohashi Y, Motoyasu A, Ando T, Moriyama K, Yorozu T. Intrathecal administration of morphine decreases persistent pain after cesarean section: A prospective observational study. PLoS One. 2016;**11**:e0155114. DOI: 10.1371/journal.pone.0155114

[115] Martinez V, Szekely B, Lemarie J, et al. The efficacy of a glial inhibitor, minocycline, for preventing persistent pain after lumbar discectomy: A randomized, double-blind, controlled study. Pain. 2013;**154**:1197-1203. DOI: 10.1016/j.pain.2013.03.028

[116] Fassoulaki A, Triga A, Melemeni A, Sarantopoulos C. Multimodal analgesia with gabapentin and local anesthetics prevents acute and chronic pain after breast surgery for cancer. Anesthesia and Analgesia. 2005;**101**:1427-1432. DOI: 10.1213/01.ANE.0000180200.11626.8E

[117] Lavand'homme P, De Kock M, Waterloos H. Intraoperative epidural analgesia combined with ketamine provides effective preventive analgesia in patients undergoing major digestive surgery. Anesthesiology. 2005;**103**:813-820

[118] Koppert W, Wehrfritz A, Korber N, et al. The cyclooxygenase isozyme inhibitors parecoxib and paracetamol reduce central hyperalgesia in humans. Pain. 2004;**108**:148-153. DOI: 10.1016/j.pain.2003.12.017

[119] Sycha T, Anzenhofer S, Lehr S, et al. Rofecoxib attenuates both primary and secondary inflammatory hyperalgesia: A randomized, double blinded, placebo controlled crossover trial in the UV-B pain model. Pain. 2005;**113**:316-322. DOI: 10.1016/j.pain.2004.11.002

[120] Buvanendran A, Kroin JS, Tuman KJ, et al. Effects of perioperative administration of a selective cyclooxygenase 2 inhibitor on pain management and recovery of function after knee replacement: A randomized controlled trial. Journal of the American Medical Association. 2003;**290**:2411-2418. DOI: 10.1001/jama.290.18.2411

[121] Meunier A, Aspenberg P, Good L. Celecoxib does not appear to affect prosthesis fixation in total knee replacement: A randomized study using radiostereometry in 50 patients. Acta Orthopaedica. 2009;**80**:46-50. DOI: 10.1080/17453670902804976

[122] Fransen M, Anderson C, Douglas J, et al. Safety and efficacy of routine postoperative ibuprofen for pain and disability related to ectopic bone formation after hip replacement surgery (HIPAID): Randomized controlled trial. BMJ. 2006;**333**:519. DOI: 10.1136/bmj.38925.471146.4F

[123] Lakdja F, Dixmerias F, Bussieres E, Fonrouge JM, Lobera A. Preventive analgesic effect of intraoperative administration of ibuprofen-arginine on postmastectomy pain syndrome. Bulletin du Cancer. 1997;**84**:259-263

[124] Romundstad L, Stubhaug A. Glucocorticoids for acute and persistent postoperative neuropathic pain: What is the evidence? Anesthesiology. 2007;**107**:371-373. DOI: 10.1097/01.anes.0000279487.27940.5c

[125] Rashiq S, Dick BD. Post-surgical pain syndromes: A review for the non-pain specialist. The Canadian Journal of Anesthesia. 2014;**61**:123-130. DOI: 10.1007/s12630-013-0072-y

Chapter 4

Acute Pain Management in Intensive Care Patients: Facts and Figures

Nissar Shaikh, Saher Tahseen, Qazi Zeesan Ul Haq,
Gamal Al-Ameri, Adel Ganaw, Arshed Chanda,
Muhammed Zubair Labathkhan and Tariq Kazi

Additional information is available at the end of the chapter

http://dx.doi.org/10.5772/intechopen.78708

Abstract

Pain is an unpleasant experience for all patients including intensive care patients; if it is not treated properly, it has deleterious effects on patients' acute and chronic well-beings. In ICU patients, it causes sympathetic stimulation leading to adverse hemodynamic effects and after discharge, these patients are at the higher risk for developing chronic pain and post-traumatic stress disorders. Apart from racial and regional factors, sleep deprivation, anxiety, and delirium increase the pain perceptions. Pain assessment is a prerequisite for adequate pain management. The ICU patients are sedated and ventilated, and assessment scales differ depending on whether the patient is able to communicate. There are different pain assessment scales for both groups of patients. The preferred mode of delivery of analgesic medication is intravenous route as intramuscular and subcutaneous route are not reliable for drug delivery in these patients. Patient and nurse controlled analgesia gives better sense of pain control. In the treatment of pain, opioids are the commonly used medications, but paracetamol, dexmedetomidine, and gabapentin are increasingly used. Newer trends are multimodal analgesia, where the combinations of analgesic medications with different mechanism of action are used. Another trend is increasing use of analgosedation; they not only control the pain but also relieve anxiety.

Keywords: pain, intensive care, pain scale, analgosedation, multimodal analgesia, opioid, paracetamol, gabapentin

1. Introduction

Pain is an unpleasant sensory and emotional experience associated with actual or potential tissue damage, or described in terms of such damage [1]. Although relieving pain is a fundamental right, still majority of the intensive care patients will experience pain sometime during their ICU stay particularly during dressing, the change of position and even at rest, and it is a great source of stress. The majority of intensive care patients may be unable to self-report their pain both verbally or with other signs because of an altered level of consciousness, the use of mechanical ventilation, or high doses of sedative agents or muscle relaxant. The incidence of significant pain is still 50% or higher in both medical and surgical ICU patients [2]. In addition to experiencing pain at rest, pain related to surgery, trauma, burns, and cancer, these patients experience procedural pain. It is ubiquitous, and inadequate treatment of procedural pain remains a significant problem for ICU patients. Nursing care procedures such as bathing, massage of back and pressure points, sheets change and repositioning are the most common painful procedures in ICU patients [2]. Vazquez et al. [3] analyzed pain intensity during 330 turnings in 96 medical surgical patients and reported significantly increased pain score between rest and turning. The bolus of analgesic was used in less than 15% of the turnings.

The adverse psychological and physiologic effects of inadequate pain control in critically ill patients are long lasting and significant. The critically ill patients have identified pain as a traumatic experience and discomforting. Recently, it is realized that more than 80% of the ICU-discharged hospitalized patients had painful memories and discomfort associated with the endotracheal tube, and 38% patients remembers pain as their worst intensive care memory even 6 months later. Granja and colleagues [4] found that 17% of patients recollect experiencing severe pain 6 months after discharge and 18% were at the risk for developing posttraumatic stress disorder (PTSD). Schelling and colleagues [5] in their follow-up study found that the patients with acute respiratory distress syndrome compared the non-ARDS patients who experience pain and other traumatic situations when they are in the intensive care unit and had a higher occurrence of chronic pain and posttraumatic stress disorders and inferior quality of life.

The stress response due to pain has serious adverse effects in intensive care patients. It increases the circulating catecholamine levels and causes arteriolar vasoconstriction, impair tissue perfusion, and reduce tissue-oxygen partial pressure [6]. Other responses triggered by pain include catabolic hypermetabolism resulting in hyperglycemia, lipolysis and breakdown of muscle to provide protein substrate [7]. These changes will impair wound healing and increase the risk of wound infection. Pain also suppresses natural killer cell activity [8, 9] and results in a decrease in the number of cytotoxic T cells, leading to a reduced neutrophil phagocytic activity [10]. Acute pain in ICU patients is a greatest risk factor for developing debilitating chronic, persistent, and neuropathic pain [11].

1.1. Pain causing organ dysfunction in the ICU patients

In the ICU, patients are in need of pain medicine for various reasons, including weaning off ventilatory support, pulmonary dysfunction and cardiac dysfunction.

1.1.1. Pulmonary complications and prolonged mechanical ventilation

Intensive care patients should be liberated from mechanical ventilation as early as possible to prevent the occurrence of ventilator-associated events. Mechanical ventilation is indirectly responsible for other medical complications such as pressure ulcers, gastric ulcers, muscular weakness and renal failure. The inadequate pain management will inhibit weaning from ventilatory support [12].

Pulmonary dysfunction is a common complication of improper pain control in postoperative upper abdominal and thoracic surgery as well as patients with abdominal pathology such as pancreatitis and bowel ischemia, and so on, it causes abdominal muscle contractions and results in a decrease in lung volumes and functional capacity The cough reflex is compromised with the abovementioned pulmonary changes and leads to retained pulmonary secretions, which complicates in the occurrence of pneumonia. Pain may induce vasoconstriction, when it is coupled with venous stasis from immobility and can lead to thrombus formation and fatal pulmonary embolism [13].

1.1.2. Cardiovascular dysfunction

Analgesia in patients with myocardial infarction or acute coronary syndrome is essentially important. Hence, morphine or other opioid analgesics are one of the components of initial therapy in these patients. Morphine reduces oxygen consumption by decreasing sympathetic activity and increases blood delivery through its vasodilatory affects [14]. Hence, it is necessary to treat the underlying cause of chest pain, but at the same time, the use of proper and adequate analgesics is recommended.

1.2. Factors modulating the pain response

Apart from racial and regional factors, anxiety, delirium, sleep deprivation and psychosocial history make ICU patients more susceptible to pain, even with the smallest stimuli. It is essential to address and minimize the following cofounding factor for pain modulation.

1.2.1. Anxiety

It is a double-edged sword, a factor causing pain and a result of pain. The intubated patients in the intensive care atmosphere have a higher anxiety and stress as they are unable to communicate and express the pain. Heightened anxiety can lead to agitation and associated with uncontrolled pain in the ICU patients. In combination with all, it can lead to patient ventilator asynchrony and difficulty in wean from the ventilator [15].

1.2.2. Delirium

It is common finding in the ICU patients, caused by environment, metabolic, intracranial, endocrine, organ failure, medication-related and respiratory conditions [15]. The ICU environment is one of the important etiologies for delirium due to the high noon level of stimulation, continuous sleep deprivation and ever-changing medical and paramedical staff. It can be challenging to appropriately assess and treat pain for patients with delirium. Few physical changes in intensive therapy environmental may decrease the occurrence of delirium. It includes having more windows, readable calendars, recognizable clocks in the ICU and to provide continuity of care. It is equally important to have a repeated and clear communication with the patient about treatments and invasive procedure plans even when patients are not able to verbally respond [15].

1.2.3. Sleep deprivation

It is an important contributing factor for increased pain response in ICU patients. In burns patients, it is a well-realized fact that if these patients do not have proper night sleep, the intensity of pain during the day time is higher [16]. Sleep deprivation in the ICU patients can result from psychological states, bright lighting, noise from ventilators and monitors, and disrupted circadian rhythms [14]. ICU patients' sleep will be improved by reducing exposure to bright light, reducing ambient noise, respecting circadian rhythms and using appropriate sedative hypnotics.

2. Pain assessment in ICU patients

It is of vital importance that the pain be assessed properly so as to manage it well. As the International Association for the Study of Pain also states, "the inability to communicate verbally does not negate the possibility that an individual is experiencing pain and is in need of appropriate pain-relieving treatment" [17]. Hence, the ICU physicians must learn to reliably detect pain, using assessment methods adapted to a patient's diminished communication capabilities. The pain assessment tools are mainly divided depending on the patient's ability to communicate or not. In later circumstances, clinicians should consider patients' behavioral reactions as surrogate measures of pain, as long as their motor function is intact [18]. Detection, quantification, and management of pain in critically ill adults are the priorities and have been the subject of research for the last two decades [19].

Pain assessments should include location, characteristics, severity, onset, progression, duration, quality, radiation, alleviating and exacerbating factors, and effects of previous therapies. Pain should be assessed by self-reporting scales in patients able to communicate, or by behavioral pain scores in patients unable to communicate. There are many self-report pain scales and behavioral pain scales developed for use in intensive care unit adult patients, which unfortunately are not always routinely used in the ICU. This self-reporting of their pain is the gold standard of pain assessment and provides the valid measurement of pain [20]. The commonly used pain intensity scales are the Numeric Rating Scale (NRS) and Visual Analogue Scale (VAS) while Behavioral Pain Scale (BPS) is considered to be an alternative tool for assessing pain in sedated and mechanically ventilated patients. The BPS assesses pain through the evaluation of facial expression, upper limb movements and compliance with mechanical ventilation. Another behavioral scale called the Critical-Care Pain Observation Tool (CPOT) may also be used.

There has been reluctance to use surrogates or individuals who make medical decisions when patients cannot do, to report patients' pain, due to their emotional attachment to these patients. They have a potential for overestimating pain. In SUPPORT study, it is concluded that surrogates can identify the patient's pain 73% of the time and accurately estimate its severity of pain 53% of the times [21].

The following pain scales will be useful in awake and cooperative patients:

http://dx.doi.org/10.5772/intechopen.78708

2.1. Visual analogue scale (VAS)

In this, the patient can see and describe the severity of pain on a scale of 0–10. Zero for no pain and 10 for maximum pain (**Figure 1**).

2.2. Numerical rating scale (NRS)

Patients rate pain by writing on a 10-point scale (**Figure 2**) (0, no pain; and 10, most severe pain).

2.3. Verbal rating scale (VRS)

In this scale, the patient can verbalize the pain in four grades. Grade 1 indicates the absence of pain, whereas severe pain is indicated by grade 4.

Pain scales and tools are used for patients unable to communicate.

2.4. Behavioral pain scale (BPS)

It is a clinical observational score depending upon the patient's facial expressions, upper limbs posturing, and tolerance of the controlled mechanical ventilation (**Table 1**). This score ranges from 3 to 12, and a score of >6 require pain management [22].

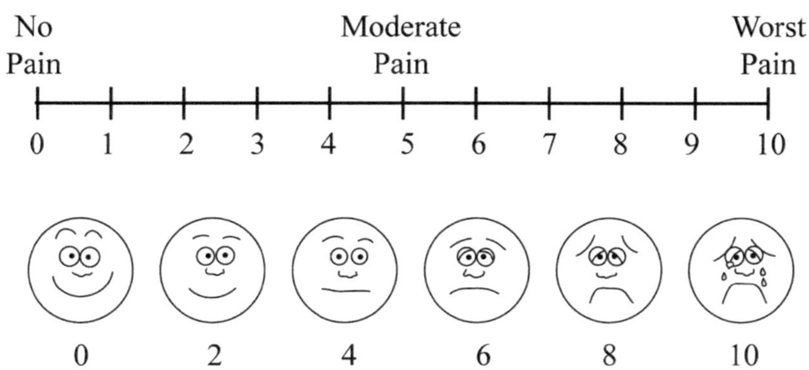

Figure 1. Visual analogue scale with its component.

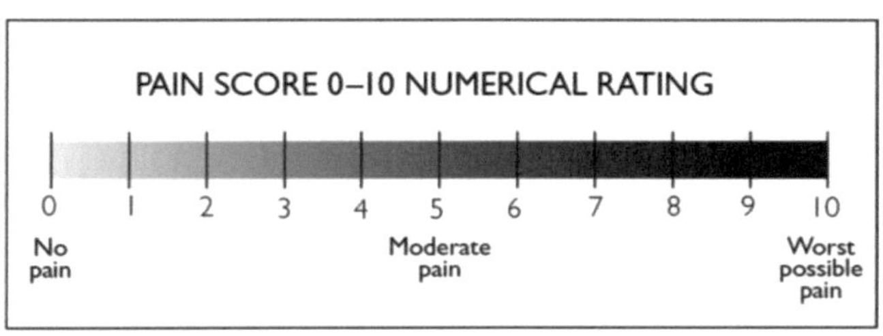

Figure 2. Numerical rating scale and its description of pain.

Facial expressions	Relaxed	1
	Partially tightened	2
	Fully tight	3
	Grimacing	4
Upper limbs	No movements	1
	Partially bent	2
	Fully bent with fingers flexion	3
	Permanently retracted	4
Compliance with mechanical ventilation	Tolerating movements	1
	Coughing but tolerating ventilation most of the time	2
	Fighting with ventilator	3
	Unable to control the ventilation	4

Table 1. Behavioral pain scale and its components.

2.5. Critical care pain observation tool (CPOT)

This pain assessment tool has four clinical components, facial expressions, body movements and muscle tension and compliance with the invasive mechanical ventilation. CPOT score ranges from 2 to 8. A score of more than 2 requires pain management.

3. Mode of analgesia administration in ICU patients

The mode of analgesic medication administration is an important factor for the pharmacologic management of pain in the ICU. Intravenous (IV) administration is more commonly the route of choice in critically ill patients because of altered GI tract function that could lead to unpredictable absorption of medication. Intravenous route is generally preferred over subcutaneous or intramuscular routes given potentially inadequate absorption due to regional hypoperfusion due to shock, subcutaneous oedema. The Fentanyl patch can be used for chronic pain relief in stable patients but not in ICUs or for acute pain relief because of the 12–24 h delay in peak serum levels.

The choice of intermittent versus continuous infusion administration depends on factors such as the frequency and severity of pain and the pharmacokinetics of the analgesic medication. The administration in bolus is associated with the variation in the peak plasma concentration, since the infusion maintains a more stable concentration but can lead to accumulation of medication in patients with renal or liver failure.

3.1. Patient-controlled analgesia (PCA)

It is an effective method for administering analgesic medication and gives patients a sense of control over their pain. Patients have autonomy on when and how much medication they receive. However, this technique requires awake and orientated patients which make use of PCA limited in ICU patients. In combination with intravenous paracetamol and pro-paracetamol, the opioid consumption is significantly less [23].

3.2. Nurse-controlled analgesia (NCA)

It is inferior to the PCA but still can be useful, as nurses can administer the analgesia quickly when required or during the procedures.

3.3. Regional (nerve blocks) and neuraxial (spinal or epidural)

Analgesia techniques are used in ICU-selected trauma patients and surgical procedures. Epidural analgesia is probably the most commonly used regional anesthetic technique in the ICU. It is more useful in critically ill postoperative thoracic, abdominal, major vascular surgery, orthopedic surgery and trauma patients. Positioning patients during catheter insertion is a challenge for using regional anesthesia in ICUs. The main disadvantages of epidural and regional analgesia are the rare but catastrophic complications such as infection, epidural hematoma formation and nerve damage, which can occur in ICU patients who have a high risk of developing these complications [24].

The combination of intravenous opioid PCA, paracetamol and regional anesthesia techniques is multimodal analgesia which decreases the total opioid analgesia consumption and hence decreasing the side effects and better patient comfort. The NCA proved to not be superior to PCA and increases the rapid response team activation.

4. Analgesic medications used in ICU patients

Opioids are the main medications used for analgesia in ICU patients due to potency, concomitant mild sedative and anxiolytic effects. It can be administered by multiple routes. The commonly use opioids include Fentanyl, Remifentanil, and Morphine. The choice of opioid and the dosing should be individualized based on potency, pharmacokinetics and pharmacodynamics, adverse effect, patient comorbidities and organ dysfunction [25].

4.1. Morphine

It is the most frequently used medication in cancer patients. It is the standard by which other opioids are compared. Morphine is directly extracted from opium poppies; it stimulates the release of histamine which produces allergic and vasodilation-induced cardiovascular instability. Initial bolus intravenous (IV) morphine 2 mg dose administered slowly over 4–5 min then can be titrated with 1–2 mg every 10–15 min till adequate analgesia is achieved. Continuous IV morphine can be administered with an initial 2–5 mg bolus dose followed by 1 mg/h. Morphine is primarily metabolized in the liver and it is excreted through kidneys. It has active metabolites; morphine-3-glucuronide and morphine-6-gluconoride. Accumulation of these metabolites in renal insufficiency can produce opioid toxicity and adverse effects such as nausea, sedation, respiratory depression myoclonus and seizures (**Table 2**) [25].

Analgesic medications	Dosage	Half-life	Main adverse effects
Morphine	2–5 mg bolus, 1–10 mg/h infusion	2–4 h	Purities, hypotension and metabolites accumulation in renal in impairment
Fentanyl	25–100 μg bolus 25–200 μg/h	2–5 h	Muscle rigidity, accumulation in hepatic impairment
Remifentanil	0.5–2 mg bolus 0.5–15 μg/kg/h	3–10 min	Bradycardia and hypotension
Dexmedetomidine	02–1.4 μg/kg/h	6 min to 3 h	Cardiac asystole, bradycardia and hypotension
Paracetamol	1 g every 6 h	2–3 h	Hypotension, liver and kidney injury

Table 2. Various opioids and non-opioid analgesic, their dosage, half-life and side effects.

4.1.1. Fentanyl

Fetany is a synthetic opioid that is 100 times more potent than morphine. It has far more lipid-soluble property than morphine and is easily taken into the CNS. Compared to morphine, it does not cause histamine release and hence no vasodilation and hypotension, making Fentanyl the preferred choice for hemodynamically unstable patients. Its intravenous onset is immediate with a short duration of 30 min to 1 h, and it is extracted though liver. Fentanyl is given IV in 25–100 μg boluses for 1–2 min and then is repeated every 10–15 min till pain is controlled. Moderate–severe pain: a loading dose of 50–200 μg intravenously followed by 25–50 μg/hr. is typically administered. Its administration for more than 5 days causes accumulation in fatty tissue, which is mobilized after the drug is stopped and may cause prolonged sedation [25].

4.1.2. Remifentanil

It is a fast-acting and an equally fast recovery drug. It is 200 times more potent than morphine. Its metabolism does not depend on the liver. Analgesia-based sedation with remifentanil is a useful option for mechanically ventilated patients, and it can be used in patients that need frequent neurological assessment. Hence, it is a drug of choice in analgosedation in ICU. It has shown a shorter duration of mechanical ventilation and quicker ICU discharge with Remifentanil compared with other opioids. It offers precise control of analgesia for painful procedures in ICU patients and has a highly predictable onset and offset, with a stable context sensitive half-time (3–10 min). Initial dose adjustment is not required for patients with impaired renal and hepatic functions. Remifentanil can be administrated in higher doses than are normally used with other opioids without concerns about accumulation and the possibility of unpredictable and/or delayed recovery. Frequently, ICU patients are managed without bolus doses, and it is recommended that remifentanil infusions should be started at 6–9 μg/kg/h and then titrated in the range dose of 0.5–15 μg/kg/h. The major adverse effects are hypotension and bradycardia (**Table 2**) [24].

4.1.3. Tramadol

It is a centrally acting opioid-like medication, acts by binding to the μ opiate receptor; it is a pure agonist and inhibits adrenaline and serotonin reuptake. The most common adverse effect includes nausea, vomiting, dizziness drowsiness, dry mouth and headache. Tramadol causes less respiratory and cardiovascular depression, euphoria and constipation. Initial bolus dosage is 100 mg. After 90 min following the initial bolus, further doses of 50 mg may be given every 30 min up to a total dose of 250 mg. Subsequent doses should be 50 or 100 mg for 4–6 h up to a total daily dose of 400 mg [24].

4.2. Non-opioid analgesic agent or adjuvants used in ICU patient

Non-opioid analgesics are use in the management of mild to moderate pain and moderate to severe pain with adjunctive opioid analgesics. The potential advantages of multimodal analgesia, which involves a combination of analgesics with different mechanisms of action, include improved analgesia with a lower opioid dose required and a decreased risk of opioid-related adverse effects [24].

4.2.1. Nonsteroidal anti-inflammatory drugs (NSAIDs)

NSAIDs have opioid-sparing effect but they are not sufficiently investigated in ICU patients. Their use in ICU patients is still controversial. The most worrying adverse effect includes gastrointestinal bleeding, renal dysfunction and inhibition of platelet function.

4.2.2. Paracetamol

It is commonly administered for the short-term treatment of mild to moderate pain and febrile critically ill patients with infection. It differs from the available opioids and NSAIDs, since paracetamol does not increase the incidence of nausea, vomiting and respiratory depression that can occur with opioids, or the platelet dysfunction, gastritis and renal toxicity that are associated with NSAIDs. It has a relatively good safety profile but there is limited information regarding IV use in critically ill patients. The study to date has described that paracetamol can cause transient abnormalities of liver function and may cause hypotension in critically ill patients. Acute liver failure is the most serious potential complication of the use of paracetamol. The key criteria for assessing potential hepatotoxicity with conventional doses of paracetamol may include hypoxic injury, altered pharmacokinetics, relative over-dosage, muscle glutathione depletion, malnutrition, dehydration, older age and alcoholism which are often seen in critically ill patients [24].

4.2.3. Prop-paracetamol

It is a prodrug form of paracetamol which is formed from the esterification of paracetamol and the carboxylic acid diethyl glycine. It has the advantage of making it more water-soluble. It is used in postoperative care and is delivered by intravenous route [23].

4.2.4. α2-agonists

The Clonidine and Dexmedetomidine are α2-adrenoceptor agonists, which provide both analgesia and sedation. Hence, they are also termed as analgosedation agents. Dexmedetomidine has eight times more affinity for α2-receptors compared with clonidine.

Dexmedetomidine infusion has been shown to reduce the prevalence and duration of confusion and delirium when compared with the use of morphine and midazolam [25].

α2-Agonists are used to improve the quality of analgesia and aid opioid rotation in opioid-tolerant individuals. The side-effect profile of both α2-agonists includes bradycardia, cardiac asystole and hypotension. Although rare, it can cause rebound hypertension and can cause withdrawal syndrome.

4.2.5. Ketamine

It is an N-methyl-aspartate antagonist, commonly used as analgosedative agent. Its use in combination with the opioid PCA reduces the opioid consumption and side effects. In combination with midazolam, ketamine provides effective analgesia in sickle cell crisis patients. Ketamine has an opioid-sparing effect and commonly used in lower dosage in burns patients. The main side effects of ketamine are tachycardia, hallucination, delirium ketotonia and increase intracranial pressure [25].

4.2.6. Magnesium

It acts through the NMDA receptors and acts as adjunct by reducing analgesic requirements without any major adverse effects, but there is no evidence that magnesium has any opioid-sparing effects in the critically ill patients [25].

4.2.7. Gabapentinoids

The Gabapentin and Pregabalin work by binding to the $\alpha 2\delta$ subunits of voltage-dependent calcium ion channels. They reduce the development of hyperalgesia and central sensitization and are useful adjuncts in the treatment of neuropathic pain.

Gabapentin compared with Carbamazepine or placebo reduces pain intensity in patients with GBS (Gillian Barrie syndrome) without increasing side effects. Gabapentinoids are used mainly in neuropathic and post-burn debridement pain. The extra advantage is that these medications are available in the enteric form and get absorbed in the duodenum; hence, one has to be careful when the patient is fed through a jeujenostomy tube. The major side effects of these medications are confusion, dizziness, ataxia and convulsions [25].

5. Few final recommending points

5.1. Hospital pain team

Consider referring complex ICU patients to the hospital pain team. It helps the patients on multimodal therapy but if still experiencing severe pain. Referral to the pain team can often lead to an increased level of support that would benefit the suffering patients, and once patients are discharged from the critical care unit, the pain team follows them to the ward [26].

5.2. Alternative therapy

The alternative medicine modalities of pain management like transcutaneous electrical nerve stimulation (TENS), acupuncture and aromatherapy have a very weak evidence base pain management in intensive care, but should be considered as the adverse-effect profile is low [25].

5.3. Reassessment

Patients must be evaluated hourly to ensure appropriate response to therapeutic interventions so that health-care providers can proactively act to relieve pain. If reassessment reveals inadequate pain control despite the initiation of therapeutic interventions, we should consider titration of medications, rotation of medications or changes in the route of administration [26].

5.4. Guidelines and protocols

These guidelines should be developed that combine a scientific basis and expert opinion. Wellness model from the World Health Organization's treatment of pain after cardiac surgery, we can see that guidelines and protocols lead to the effective management of post-cardiac surgery pain. If we look at the complexity of ICU pain, we need to have organized protocols to help us care for these patients. The examination of published literature reviews and evidence-based guidelines can facilitate the development of institution-specific guidelines.

5.5. Clinical pathways

It provides a consistent and repeatable time line for planning individualized patient care. The pathway details the precise course of the patient, including multidisciplinary elements. It includes history, examination, diagnostics and treatment and incorporates pre-emptive treatment for procedures as well as management of chronic pain issues [26].

5.6. Checklists

It is a way to verify that clinical pathways or tasks are completed and it is a good way to ensure that pathways or tasks are followed. It helps in errors prevention [26].

5.7. Daily goals

Daily goals highlighting by white board, electronic reminders to all members of the multidisciplinary team can access the plan and ensure that the patient is being treated from all perspectives [26].

6. Conclusions

Intensive care unit (ICU) patients are at the higher risk of pain and they are having pain even while resting. If pain is not adequately treated, it leads to adverse effect and increases the chances of chronic pain and posttraumatic stress disorders in these patients. In ICU patient, anxiety, delirium and sleep deprivation increase the sensitivity to pain. The organ dysfunctions in these patients will decrease the potency of analgesic medication and increase the toxicity. Pain assessment is the basic essential factor in adequate management of pain. The different pain scales are used depending on their abilities to communicate. The commonly used analgesic medication in ICU patients is opioids but there is an increased use of multimodal analgesia and analgosedation approach obvious reasons. In the management of pain in ICU patients, the involvement of pain management teams, the use of clinical pathway, guidelines and protocols may have better impacts.

Author details

Nissar Shaikh[1]*, Saher Tahseen[1], Qazi Zeesan Ul Haq[1], Gamal Al-Ameri[1], Adel Ganaw[1], Arshed Chanda[1], Muhammed Zubair Labathkhan[1] and Tariq Kazi[2]

*Address all correspondence to: nissatfirdous99@gmail.com

1 Surgical Intensive Care Unit: Hamad Medical Corporation, Weill Cornell Medical Collage in Doha, Doha, Qatar

2 Medical Intensive Care Unit: Hamad Medical Corporation, Doha, Qatar

References

[1] Barr J, Puntillo K, Ely EW, Gélinas C, Dasta JF, et al. Clinical practice guidelines for the Management of Pain, agitation, and delirium in adult patients in the intensive care unit. Critical Care Medicine. 2013;**41**:264-306

[2] de Jong A, Molinari N, De Lattre S. Decreasing severe pain and serious adverse events while moving intensive care unit patients: A prospective interventional study (the NURSE-DO project). Critical Care. 2013;**17**:R74

[3] Vazquez M, Pardavila MI, Lucia M, Aguado Y, Margall MA, Asiain MC. Pain assessment in turning procedures for patients with invasive mechanical ventilation. Nursing in Critical Care. 2011;**16**:178-185

[4] Granja C, Gomes E, Amaro A, et al. JMIP study group: Understanding posttraumatic stress disorder-related symptoms after critical care: The early illness amnesia hypothesis. Critical Care Medicine. 2008;**36**:2801-2809

[5] Schelling G, Stoll C, Haller M, et al. Health-related quality of life and posttraumatic stress disorder in survivors of the acute respiratory distress syndrome. Critical Care Medicine. 1998;**26**:651-659

[6] Akça O, Melischek M, Scheck T, et al. Postoperative pain and subcutaneous oxygen tension. Lancet. 1999;**354**:41-42

[7] Hedderich R, Ness TJ. Analgesia for trauma and burns. Critical Care Clinics. 1999; **15**:167-184

[8] Beilin B, Shavit Y, Hart J, et al. Effects of anesthesia based on large versus small doses of fentanyl on natural killer cell cytotoxicity in the perioperative period. Anesthesia and Analgesia. 1996;**82**:492-497

[9] Pollock RE, Lotzová E, Stanford SD. Mechanism of surgical stress impairment of human perioperative natural killer cell cytotoxicity. Archives of Surgery. 1991;**126**:338-342

[10] Peterson PK, Chao CC, Molitor T, et al. Stress and pathogenesis of infectious disease. Reviews of Infectious Diseases. 1991;**13**:710-720

[11] Puntillo KA, Miaskowski C, Summer G. Pain. In: Carrieri-Kohlman V, Lindsey AM, West CM, editors. Pathophysiological Phenomena in Nursing: Human Responses to Illness. 3rd ed. St. Louis, MO: Saunders; 2003. pp. 235-255

[12] Marino PL. Analgesia and sedation. In: Marino PL, Sutin KM, editors. The ICU Book. 3rd ed. Philadelphia, PA: Lippincott Williams & Wilkins; 2007. pp. 885-907

[13] Desai PM. Pain management and pulmonary dysfunction. Critical Care Clinics. 1999; **15**:151-166

[14] American Heart Association. 2005 American Heart Association guidelines for cardiopulmonary resuscitation and emergency cardiovascular care part 8: Stabilization of the patient with acute coronary syndrome. Circulation;**2005**(112):89-110

[15] Szokol JW, Verdin JS. Anxiety, delirium and pain in the intensive care unit. Critical Care Clinics. 2001;**17**:821-841

[16] Raymond I, Nielsen TA, Lavigne G, Manzini C, Choiniere M. Quality of sleep and its daily relationship to pain intensity in hospitalized adult burn patients. Pain. 2001;**92**:381-388

[17] International association for the study of pain. IASP taxonomy. Available at: http://www.iasp-pain.org/AM/Template.cfm?Section=Pain_Defi

[18] Anand KJ, Craig KD. New perspectives on the definition of pain. Pain. 1996;**67**:3-6 discussion 209

[19] Puntillo KA. Pain experiences of intensive care unit patients. Heart & Lung. 1990; **19**:526-533

[20] Hamill-Ruth RJ, Marohn ML. Evaluation of pain in critically ill patients. Critical Care Clinics. 1999;**15**:35-54

[21] Desbiens NA, Mueller-Rizner N. How well do surrogates assess the pain of seriously ill patients? Critical Care Medicine. 2000;**28**:1347-1352

[22] Payen J, Bru O, Bosson J, et al. Assessing pain in critically ill sedated patients by using a behavioural pain scale. Critical Care Medicine. 2001;**29**:2258-2263

[23] shaikh N, Kettern MA, Ahmed AHA, Louon A. Morphine sparing effect of Proparacetamol in surgical and trauma intensive care. The Middle East Journal of Emergency medicine. 2006;**6**:28-30

[24] Višnja Nesek A et al. Pain management in critically ill patients. Periodicum Biologorum. 2015;**57**:61

[25] Narayanan M, Venkataraju A, Jennings J. Analgesia in intensive care: part 1. BJA Education. 2016;**16**:72-78

[26] https://www.practicalpainmanagement.com/resources/managing-pain-intensive-care-units; downloaded on 17th Feb 2018

Chapter 5

Pain Management for Pregnant Women in the Opioid Crisis Era

Ahmed Zaghw, Mohamed Koronfel,
Edward Podgorski, Sara Siddiqui, Arif Valliani,
Arunabha Karmakar and Jaffar Khan

Additional information is available at the end of the chapter

http://dx.doi.org/10.5772/intechopen.79333

Abstract

Acute and chronic pain management during pregnancy, after delivery and even during lactation are challenging even for experienced physicians. This chapter intends to cover pregnancy-induced physiological changes in relation to pain conditions. It also covers the most common pain disorders in pregnancy and provides a comprehensive summary of the pharmacological and non-pharmacological options for pain management in pregnancy. Additionally, pain management in context of opioid abuse will also be covered, as high prevalence of opioid prescription is linked to the very poor maternal and fetal outcomes. The possibility of maternal opioid abuse and fetal opioid withdrawal should be known to all physicians, given its rising trends. Multimodal protocols and opioid sparing strategies are highly essential for safe pain management during pregnancy and have been discussed. This chapter is intended to be a fast and detailed review for residents, pain fellows, and physicians who seek pain control in pregnant women.

Keywords: pain management during pregnancy, pregnancy related musculoskeletal pain, non-pharmacological pain management, opioid crisis, opioid use disorder, neonatal abstinence syndrome

1. Introduction

Pain during pregnancy is not necessarily limited to labor pain and includes musculoskeletal, urological, neuropathic, and psychosocial pain. This can pose a diagnostic and management challenges, especially in terms of medication selection. If left untreated, it can lead to anxiety, depression, and even physical disability. Pain can persist postpartum with severe symptoms in 10% of patients and can sometimes last for more than 10 years after delivery [1]. There are multiple barriers to effective pain management in pregnancy. In addition to the complex and multifactorial nature of pain, there is a worldwide misconception that acute musculoskeletal pain during pregnancy is a normal physiological consequence that should be coped with. There is also fear of undesirable pharmacological effects of pain medicines on the fetus that prevent patients from pursuing treatment options.

Another challenge is the ongoing opioid crisis. Progressive increase in opioid prescription and lack of familiarity with non-pharmacological pain management or multimodal protocols have led to a sharp increase in opioid abuse, admission to rehabilitation facilities, and increased overall maternal and fetal morbidity and mortality [2].

2. Physiological changes in pregnancy affecting pain

Pain occurring in pregnancy could be a result of mechanical and/or biochemical changes arising from changing physiology. The average pregnant woman gains 10–18 kg of weight (an approximate of 20% increase from baseline), doubling the mechanical load on axial joints and ligaments [3, 4]. The core muscles responsible for core stabilization and balance are stressed as well. The gravid uterus stretches the abdominal muscles and pelvic floor muscles. There is an upward shift of the center of gravity leading to some compensatory hyperlordosis with stretching of lower back muscles, significant anterior pelvic tilt with rotation of the pelvis on the femur, and increased use of hip extensors and abductors. There is also more head flexion and drooping of the shoulders [5]. Enlarged breasts and malposition during breastfeeding could also lead to thoracic kyphosis.

Hormonally induced structural changes include increased ligament and joint laxity, decreased bone density and weaker collagen, all of which have been associated with back pain [6, 7]. The Relaxin hormone is secreted from the placental decidua and corpus luteum to increase the myometrium relaxation and cervical softening by altering the matrix metalloproteinase and glycosaminoglycan compositions [8]. While the correlation of Relaxin hormone level with pain has been inconsistent, it can contribute to joint and ligament laxity and symphysis pubis dilation [7]. There is fluid gain of 2–3 l, which are locally entrapped in legs and ankles which in addition to global water retention contributes to joint stress [9]. This further contributes to joint stress. Improper joint loading can persist in the postpartum period due to continued ligament laxity and core muscle weakness. The net effect is low back pain (LBP) and pelvic girdle pain (PGP).

3. Non-labor chronic pain

Acute and chronic pains are very common in pregnancy, with an incidence of at least 60% for LBP and 20% for PGP. Chronic non-labor pain is any subjective unpleasant sensory experience, both physically and emotionally, with actual tissue damage not relating to obstetric origin for more than 6 months. Some authors accept a 3-month timeframe if pure central neuromodulation has been documented [10]. Chronic pain has been associated with poor academic achievement, increased job loss, disability, anxiety, depression, sexual dysfunction and reduction in relationship satisfaction. These collectively contribute to a lower quality of life (QOL) [11]. Chronic pain guidelines classify chronic pain into pain with a specifically identifiable pathology (such as infection or malignancy) for which there is specific treatment or pain with non-specific pathology. Non-specific pain could be somatic, visceral, neuropathic, psychosocial, or combined. (**Table 1**) summarizes the type of chronic pain in pregnant women.

Somatic	**Musculoskeletal**	Pelvic floor dysfunction Spondylosis Myofascial syndrome—fibromyalgia
Visceral	**Gynecologic**	Endometriosis (most common) Pelvic adhesive/congestion syndrome **Infections**: Tuberculous salpingitis—chronic PID **Malignancy**: Gynecologic malignancy **Mechanical**: Prolapse of pelvic contents Adnexal cysts—cervical stenosis
	Urological	Congenital: Urethral diverticulum **Malignancy**: Bladder neoplasm **Infection**: Nongynecologic—interstitial cystitis Recurrent UTI—urethritis **Stones**: (nephrolithiasis/urolithiasis)
	Gastrointestinal	**Inflammatory**: Inflammatory bowel disease Diverticulitis—colitis—celiac sprue **Malignancy**: Colon neoplasm **Functional**: Irritable bowel syndrome Constipation
Neuropathic	• Herniated disk—cauda equina syndrome • Neuralgia—nerve impingement	
Psychosocial	• Prior or current physical or sexual abuse • Depression—somatization disorder • Substance abuse	

Table 1. Chronic pain conditions in pregnant women.

3.1. Musculoskeletal pain

Musculoskeletal pain is any pain that originates from muscles, tendons, or ligaments. Back pain and pelvic pain are among the most common types of chronic musculoskeletal pain in pregnancy [5]. Other less common types are cervical, thoracic, rib, abdominal wall, and chest wall pain. Acute musculoskeletal pain directly after labor could be due to sacral stress fracture, coccydynia (from coccygeal fracture, dislocation, or contusion), perineal tear after traumatic vaginal delivery, or symphysis pubis pain (from contusion or symphysis separation).

3.1.1. Lower back pain

Lower back pain (**LBP**) is any pain occurring between the 12th rib and the gluteal fold. **LBP** commonly occurs at lumbar spine level L4-5 and is believed to be a combination of mechanical strains, muscles weakness, joint laxity, and connective tissue edema without any identifiable etiology on imaging studies [12]. Less common causes are myofascial pain, lumbar disc herniations, and true sciatica. Magnetic resonance studies did not show any difference in the incidence of asymptomatic disc bulge or herniation in pregnant women compared with non-pregnant women [12].

3.1.2. Pelvic girdle pain

Pelvic girdle pain (**PGP**) is any pain occurring between the posterior iliac crest and gluteal fold down to the symphysis pubis. Also called lumbopelvic pain, it is the second most common pregnancy-related musculoskeletal complaint after LBP; however, it is even more disabling. **PGP** is classified into four categories: unilateral sacroiliac syndrome, bilateral sacroiliac syndrome, symphysiolysis (separation of the pubis), and pelvic girdle syndrome (pain in all three pelvic joint regions, namely the two sacroiliac joints and the pubis). The sacroiliac joint (**SIJ**) is the most common source of pelvic girdle pain in pregnancy [20], followed by pelvic floor muscle dysfunction, which is prevalent in 50% of pregnant women with pelvic pain. MRI studies have reported the pregnancy-induced SIJ changes to be SIJ-bone marrow edema (BME), joint fluid accumulation, capsulitis, enthesitis, and subchondral sclerosis [13].

3.1.3. Risk for musculoskeletal pain

While mechanical strain can occur routinely in pregnancy, musculoskeletal pain development is not universal. Risk factors include multiparity, preexisting joint disorders, obesity, and depression. LBP progressively increases with each trimester; however, it has a favorable postpartum course as the pain resolves at least in 80% of patients. Unfortunately, 20% of patients still report pain up to 3 years after delivery. The underlying etiology, severity of the symptoms and degree of anatomical changes (such as exaggerated symphysis widening and pelvic asymmetry) determine the intrapartum and postpartum prognosis. Bone marrow distension and joint capsular edema usually resolve after delivery, but autoimmune-related joint conditions such as multiple sclerosis and rheumatoid arthritis usually flare up in the postpartum period after the cessation of pregnancy-induced autoimmune modulation [14, 15].

http://dx.doi.org/10.5772/intechopen.79333

3.2. Management of musculoskeletal pain

3.2.1. History and physical examination

A comprehensive and structured history is the first step for pain management in any patient. This includes:

- Detailed nature of the pain (onset, course, duration, alleviating and aggravating factors, and radiation)
- Functional limitations, other persistent pain conditions
- History of other comorbidities (e.g., diabetes mellitus, autoimmune diseases)
- History of illicit drug abuse
- Social and family support, coping mechanisms
- Alarming neurological signs as urinary retention (with overflow incontinence), bladder or bowel incontinence, saddle anesthesia, loss of anal sphincter tone, major motor weakness in lower extremities, and fever
- Any suspicion of infection, fracture, or malignancy should be investigated, and tertiary neurosurgical referral is warranted urgently

The **general** examination starts with inspection of the skin, spine, and pelvic contour; palpation of surrounding muscles, SIJ, and facet joints for tenderness; and determination of gait pattern. In SIJ and facet joint arthropathy, there is localized tenderness over the affected joints with increased pain on axial rotation. Discogenic pain radiates to back of the thigh and worsens with the flexion of the spine.

Special physical tests for back pain are designed to provoke reproducible pain during the joint action with high specificity and sensitivity. Thus, they can be relied upon for preliminary diagnosis and follow up. These include active straight leg raise (ASLR) test for LBP and Patrick's Faber test for PGP, pubic symphysis palpation and modified Trendelenburg's test for symphysis pubis pain, posterior pelvic pain provocation (PPPP) test for posterior pelvic pain, and long dorsal sacroiliac ligament (LDL) palpation for SIJ pain. Physical examination can be helpful in identifying symptomatic herniated disc and its alarming signs. However, it is not very helpful to definitely locate the anatomic source of other non-discogenic pain even after imaging studies [16]. In general, a single physical test is less useful than combined tests for clinical decision, thus combined clusters of physical examinations are recommended for better test reliability [17].

3.2.2. Laboratory investigations for musculoskeletal pain

There are no recommendations for routine laboratory investigations for musculoskeletal pain unless there is suspicion of infection or malignancy. Consider CBC, ESR, and CRP in suspected malignancy, or thyroid assay if hypothyroidism is suspected, and any blood investigations according to provisional diagnosis.

3.2.3. Radiological investigations for musculoskeletal pain

There are no recommendations for routine radiological scans in acute or chronic back pain without warning signs. The European guidelines for diagnosis and treatment of PGP recommends against routine imaging for musculoskeletal pain during pregnancy. No significant differences were found in short- or long-term pain outcomes or functional recovery outcomes between immediate imaging versus routine care in patients with LBP in the absence of warning signs [18]. Due to poor sensitivity in detecting the early degenerative stages of SIJ arthritis, computed tomography (CT) and conventional radiography are not recommended. MRI is more favorable as a diagnostic alternative as there is no exposure to radiation and it is more reliable in discriminating changes around joints and ligaments. MRI is recommended for LBP, PGP and SIJ pain only in case of traumatic injuries, tumor, ankylosing spondylitis, and alarming signs [19].

3.2.4. Treatment of musculoskeletal pain

Treatment of musculoskeletal pain should be in a structured, multimodal approach. This involves the combination of non-pharmacological and pharmacological options. Surgical intervention is only reserved for emergency situations (acute disc herniation and cauda equina syndrome).

Non-pharmacological modalities include physical exercise and other alternatives such as massage, acupuncture, relaxation techniques, and chiropractic care. Physical exercise helps strengthen muscles of the back, abdomen, and pelvic floor to maintain core stability and augment joint stabilization.

The first line pharmacological treatment for mild pain is a short course of analgesics such as acetaminophen. NSAIDs can be used for no more than 2 days at a time, and it is contraindicated in the third trimester and preferably to be avoided in first trimester. Opioids should also be avoided throughout the pregnancy. In chronic pain studies, prolonged opioid use did not show any benefit in functional outcome or reduction of pain intensity [20]. Moreover, it can increase pain sensitivity in the long run. Most medical societies agree about the judicious use of opioid in chronic pain, as summarized in **Table 2**.

3.3. Migraine

The incidence of new-onset migraine during pregnancy is around 2–3%. However, it is more common for pregnant women to have a prior history of migraine. Fortunately, severity and frequency of migraine symptoms reduce by 43–86%, mostly during the first trimester. Sumatriptan is considered safe and is recommended by the European Federation of Neurological Societies as abortive migraine therapy [21]. It is considered non-teratogenic and, despite the theoretical vasoconstrictor effect, no vascular malformations were reported. However, it has been associated with uterine atony and peripartum hemorrhage [22]. Ergot derivatives are contraindicated during pregnancy and lactation due to their high teratogenic

Recommendation 1: **"Strong Evidence"**	**Optimization** of non-opioid pharmacotherapy and non-pharmacological therapy **before** trial of opioids.
Recommendation 2: "Weak Evidence"	In persistent problematic pain despite optimized non-opioid therapy, **Opioid trial can be started** if, 1. Chronic non-cancer pain 2. No current/past substance use 3. No active psychiatric disorders
Recommendation 3: **"Strong Evidence"**	In Patients with current substance use disorder, **Opioid is strongly not recommended.** Substance use disorder as alcohol abuse and dependence, and narcotic abuse and dependence should be addressed by physician.
Recommendation 4: "Weak Evidence"	In Patients with current active psychiatric disorder, **Optimization of** psychiatric disorder **is strongly recommended before Opioid trial.** as long as **1.** Optimal non-opioid, non-pharmacological therapy for chronic non-cancer pain has been achieved.
Recommendation 5: **"Strong Evidence"**	In **long term** opioid for non-cancer chronic pain patients should be **restricted to less 90 mg morphine equivalents** daily rather than no upper limit or a higher limit on dosing.
Recommendation 6: "Weak Evidence"	Starting **opioid** for non-cancer chronic pain patients should be **restricted to less 50 mg morphine equivalents** daily rather than no upper limit or a higher limit on dosing.
Recommendation 7: "Weak Evidence"	**Opioids rotation** and **tapering** for current opioid users in case of **1.** Persistent non-cancer pain or 2. Adverse events *"Rotation is parallel with the goal of dose reduction"*
Recommendation 8: "Weak Evidence"	**Tapering opioids** to the **lowest effective dose** with the aim to **discontinuation.**
Recommendation 9: **"Strong Evidence"**	**Multidisciplinary team** (MDT) program is highly recommended for patients using opioids and experiencing serious adverse events. *"MDT is not limited to a primary care physician, a nurse, a pharmacist, a physical therapist, a chiropractor, a kinesiologist, an occupational therapist, an addiction specialist, a psychiatrist, and a psychologist"*

Table 2. Summary of the 2017 Canadian Guidelines for Opioids for Chronic Non-Cancer Pain.

risk, uterine vasoconstriction, low birth weight, preterm contractions and miscarriage, and even convulsions in breastfed infant [23]. Beta-blockers are the first line prophylactic option during lactation and are considered safe during pregnancy. Angiotensin-converting enzyme inhibitors are contraindicated because of their nephrotoxicity and prematurity risk [22]. Non-pharmacological options include relaxation techniques, acupuncture, biofeedback, and behavioral cognitive therapy. Acetaminophen is ideal as first add-on medication. If acetaminophen fails, sumatriptan or NSAIDs could be added to the regimen based on clinical assessment and potential risk to the fetus.

3.4. Neuropathic pain

Causes of neuropathic pain in pregnancy include carpal tunnel syndrome, meralgia paresthetica, low intercostal nerve compression, and the pain of a previous cesarean section wound scar. Physiological water retention, obesity, and diabetes are contributory factors for neuropathic pain. Pregnancy-related carpal tunnel syndrome (PRCTS) is as prevalent as 43%, as confirmed by nerve conduction studies [24]. It manifests as pain and numbness in the distribution of the median nerve with progressive worsening at night. CTS usually subsides by conservative treatment and night splints. Physical therapy, infiltration of local anesthetic, and slow-release steroids could be added. Surgical decompression is rarely required and is reserved only for severe cases with motor neuropathy [25]. Differential diagnosis includes De-Quervain tendinopathy which presents with pain, swelling, and tenderness along the radial aspect of the wrist. Meralgia paresthetica is mononeuropathy of the lateral femoral cutaneous nerve (LFCN) which presents as tingling and numbness in the anterolateral aspect of the thigh.

4. Summary of non-labor pain management algorithm

A structured, multimodal approach is the essence of management of NLP. It is essential to set realistic goals based on functional status rather than chasing a pain score of zero. The impact of setting realistic goals of pain management has been shown to produce more patient satisfaction, better psychological well-being, higher quality of life and reduced anxiety [26, 27]. On the other hand, a patient feeling her pain is poorly controlled leads to more disability, increased pain intensity, anxiety, and depression [28, 29].

Non-pharmacological therapies are very valuable as they augment pain relief and minimize the utilization of drugs. These benefits are welcomed by pregnant women who often have concerns about medications and their side effects. Activity modifications, physical exercise, and a physiotherapy program have been shown to be effective in pain reduction in comparison with standard care. The additive benefit of combining different approaches such as adding acupuncture to stabilization exercises, has been proven in different studies. Pelvic belt bracing has been shown to improve SIJ stability by decreasing joint laxity and sagittal rotation by 19% [30].

5. Summary of pharmacological management

5.1. Teratogenicity and toxicity

Agents that are toxic and cause birth defects are known as teratogens [31]. During fetal development, teratogens impart their effect mostly during the time of organogenesis which begins in the third week of gestation. The severity of malformation depends on many factors, including type of teratogenic agent, dose and duration of exposure, time period of gestation, and

Category A: No fetal risk in human studies	
Category B: No fetal risk in animal studies, but no human studies	
Category C: Harmful fetal risk in animal studies, but no human studies	
Category D: Harmful fetal risk in human studies, but use is acceptable in serious situation	
Category X: Harmful fetal risk in both animal and human studies.	

Table 3. FDA classification for safety of medications in pregnancy.

maternal and fetal health prior to the exposure. Teratogenicity can be caused by fetal cell death leading to spontaneous abortion, impaired cellular functions, or placental toxicity [31].

The US Food and Drug Administration (FDA) classification for safety of medications in pregnancy is shown in "**Table 3**" [32].

5.2. Opioid medications

Codeine, hydrocodone, oxycodone, and propoxyphene are currently among the most commonly prescribed opioid agents in the United States [33]. Opioid medications should not be considered as a homogenous class of medications regarding its maternal and fetal effects, as some subclass are safer than the others. Evidence is still inconclusive regarding the relationship of opioid with poor fetal growth, preterm birth, and birth defects as most of the studies were biased with a lot of confounders. The general recommendation is that opioid usage should be avoided or minimized during pregnancy and should never be considered as a first line option. Usage during early pregnancy could be associated with neural tube defects and heart defects, and during late pregnancy, with neonatal abstinence syndrome (NAS) and neonatal respiratory distress syndrome. All opioid medications are classified as Class C (uncertain safety, no human studies; animal studies show an adverse effect).

Fentanyl patches seem to be safe, but there is still a risk of withdrawal. Methadone is associated with neonatal morbidity, such as preterm birth (<32 weeks of gestation), low birth weight, decreased head circumference, jaundice, thrombocytosis, arrhythmia, and admission to the neonatal intensive care unit [34, 35]. Codeine is classified as category C by the FDA [36]. It is neither teratogenic nor associated with congenital malformation. However, there have been reports of postpartum hemorrhage if it was taken near the end of pregnancy. Moreover, it could be rapidly metabolized into morphine, by CYP450 enzymes leading to a significant risk of fetal opioid toxicity during lactation [37]. Tramadol is classified as a category C medication. It has a risk of withdrawal with high maternal dosing [32]. It is not recommended to discontinue it during breastfeeding as only trace amounts cross into the breast milk.

The morphine equivalent daily dosage (MEDD) is a mean of calculating the daily cumulative intake of any opioid-related drugs. The aim is to reduce the risk of overdose, especially in chronic opioid use. Evidence has shown that there is no single dosage threshold below which overdose risk could be avoided, but opioid dosages of <50 MEDD/day (mg/day) would likely reduce the risk of fatal overdose.

5.3. Non-opioid analgesic medications

5.3.1. Acetaminophen (paracetamol)

Acetaminophen is widely used as an analgesic. In the USA, 65–70% of women used acetaminophen during pregnancy [38]. It has no known maternal adverse outcomes or fetal congenital defects as confirmed by analysis of registries [39]. Despite the reports about increased risk of attention deficit hyperactive disorder (ADHD) in children if used for over 6 weeks, the evidence was inconclusive according to the latest FDA warning [40].

5.3.2. Non-steroidal anti-inflammatory agents

Non-steroidal anti-inflammatory agents (NSAIDs) such as Ibuprofen, Naproxen, Diclofenac, and Celecoxib are very commonly prescribed for analgesia. It was reported that 18–25 and 4% of the USA pregnant women are exposed to over-the-counter (OTC) Ibuprofen, and Naproxen respectively [38]. In the third trimester, NSAIDs are linked with premature closure of the ductus arteriosus and development of pulmonary hypertension in a fetus. At high doses, NSAIDs decrease renal perfusion in fetus and lead to oligohydramnios. Despite NSAIDs being Category B drugs before the third trimester, it is generally recommended to be avoided as in the first trimester there is risk of miscarriage and in the third trimester there is a risk of oligohydramnios and ill effect on fetal circulation. Furthermore, NSAIDs are associated with a delay in onset of labor and increase in duration.

5.3.3. Aspirin

Aspirin is not commonly used to treat pain or fever in pregnancy. It is associated with neonatal hemorrhage, IUGR, gastroschisis and perinatal death. Similar to NSAIDs, they delay onset of labor and increase labor duration. An increased risk of bleeding during delivery has also been reported. Low-dose Aspirin (81 mg) is considered safe and is commonly given with heparin in conditions with recurrent miscarriage and in women with antiphospholipid syndrome [41].

5.4. Psychotropic medications

Psychotropic drugs are medications that affect mood, cognitive function or any other mental process [42]. These include antidepressants, benzodiazepines, antiepileptic agents and antipsychotics. Most of the safety profiles and recommendations for using these drugs are based on retrospective observational studies in pregnant patients with underlying psychiatric or mood disorders (such as bipolar or depression or anxiety) and are thus liable to bias and confounding. Some medications are well known to cause significant congenital malformations, such as Valproate, Carbamazepine, Lithium, and Lamotrigine. Therefore, they must be avoided in pregnancy. Most of other drugs are debated in their fetal outcome. In general, the risk-benefit ratio should be weighed, and the lowest dose should be applied.

5.4.1. Antidepressants

Patients with chronic pain commonly experience depression. Selective serotonin receptor inhibitors (SSRIs) and tricyclic antidepressants (TCAs) are widely used as antidepressants and also as adjuvant therapy for chronic pain. SSRIs have been the most commonly studied antidepressants in pregnancy and include Citalopram, Escitalopram, Fluoxetine, Fluvoxamine, Paroxetine, and Sertraline. There is little information about other SSRIs. Majority of studies report that SSRIs are not teratogenic; however, some consider them as low-risk teratogens as due to there has been associated increase, albeit minimal, in cardiac congenital anomalies in the form of small ventricular defects that spontaneously close in childhood [43, 44]. The use of SSRIs minimally increases the risk of antepartum and postpartum hemorrhage. There has been no increase in the risk of spontaneous abortions, perinatal deaths, or hypertensive disorders of pregnancy. Peripartum fetal exposure is not believed to be associated with postpartum withdrawal or toxicity symptoms in the neonate. Case reports that had reported an association were confounded by other psychotropic medications [45]. Among SSRIs, sertraline has the safest profile as its low levels in blood and breast milk [46].

TCAs are believed to be generally nonteratogenic except Clomipramine as reported by most studies. All drugs in this class could increase the risk of spontaneous abortion, hypertensive disorders of pregnancy, postpartum hemorrhage and transient fetal withdrawal symptoms [47]. There is still limited information and less usage of antidepressants drugs other than SSRIs, such as Selective Serotonin Norepinephrine Reuptake Inhibitors (SNRIs) and atypical antidepressants like Mirtazapine and Buspirone.

5.4.2. Benzodiazepines

A majority of studies report benzodiazepines to be nonteratogenic. Even the few conflicting reports showed that the incidence of minor anomalies such as cleft palate is only minimally increased compared with the general population. Perinatal usage increases the risk of low birth weight, preterm labor and spontaneous abortion. Moreover, peripartum exposure is associated with withdrawal and toxicity symptoms [48].

5.4.3. Antiepileptic agents

Antiepileptic drugs are now commonly used in pain management, particularly for the treatment of neuropathic pain such as, trigeminal neuralgia, diabetic neuropathy, post-herpetic neuralgia, post-stroke pain, phantom limb pain and pain after spinal cord injuries. Majority of studies have reported significant fetal morbidity due to in-utero exposure that including major anomalies like neural tube defects, congenital heart abnormalities, and urinary tract defects, skeletal abnormalities, cleft palate and impaired cognitive and motor development [49, 50]. Pregabalin, which is very commonly prescribed for chronic neuropathic pain, has a better safety profile than other antiepileptics. However, it is still associated with a higher risk for malformation than in the general population [51].

5.4.4. Antipsychotic agents

In recent times, Olanzapine, the atypical antipsychotic, has been gaining popularity in chronic pain management. A majority of studies report Olanzapine as nonteratogenic and not associated with spontaneous abortions or major congenital malformations. Nevertheless, it has been associated with an increase in birth weight [52].

6. Non-pharmacological management

6.1. Physical therapy

Physical therapy has been one of the cornerstones of chronic pain treatment, replacing the original approach of rest. Activities are aimed at restoring flexibility, strength, and endurance, as well as reducing the severity of chronic pain through modulation of the biochemical processes within the body [30, 53]. Numerous physical therapy programs exist (e.g., aerobic, yoga, tai chi, strength, pilates, flexibility, and range of motion), and each one differs in frequency, intensity, and design. Despite the high utilization of physical therapy and several studies that have demonstrated its benefits in chronic pain, the effectiveness of physical therapy is unclear and current high-quality evidence to support such claims are lacking [53–56]. Absolute contraindications are myocardial infarction, ongoing unstable angina, and severe aortic stenosis [56]. Adverse effects of physical therapy are rare with musculoskeletal injury being the most common. Other potential adverse events include pain exacerbations, soreness, rhabdomyolysis, dehydration, hypo- and hyperthermia, and cardiac and respiratory events [57]. Importantly, neither the AHA nor the systemic reviews site pregnancy as an absolute or relative contraindication to physical therapy. Currently, the consensus is that the potential benefits of physical activity in pain relief, and improved quality of life outweigh its risks. For maximum effectiveness and minimum adverse effects, the evidence suggests that supervised and structured program schedules are superior to self-supervised and varying program schedules [53]. Moreover, adding a specifically tailored training to a standard physical exercise has less disability and more functional recovery at 2 years postpartum in comparison with physical exercise alone [58].

6.2. Acupuncture

Acupuncture is a technique where needles or other modalities are used to stimulate predetermined locations throughout the body to promote the flow of 'Qi' and rebalance the body's energy. Although the practice originated in China thousands of years ago, the specific mechanism of action has yet to be uncovered. Current theories suggest that acupuncture boosts the body's intrinsic neuropeptide pathways, including endogenous opioids. However, these effects appear to be short term and do not explain the longer term benefits of acupuncture [59]. Due to the heterogeneity of acupuncture techniques, outcomes are hard to study and compare. A few studies have shown benefits, including several randomized controlled trials which demonstrated acupuncture to be an effective alternative to pharmacologic treatment [60]. However, these studies focused on labor-related pain and not chronic pain during pregnancy. In addition, meta-analyses have suggested that any superiority of acupuncture over sham acupuncture is not clinically significant [61, 62]. The literature does not suggest any absolute contraindications to acupuncture, but relative contraindications are similar to other needling techniques used for the treatment of pain. The incidence of serious adverse risks is rare (estimated to be 0.05 per 10,000 treatments) and is generally associated with poorly trained or unlicensed acupuncturists. The two most common adverse risks reported in one study were needling pain (3.3%) and hematoma (3.2%). Other risks include bruising, syncope, exacerbation of symptoms, paresthesia, infection, retained needle, and damage to surrounding tissues [63]. Two studies have commented on the adverse effects of acupuncture during pregnancy, and both suggest that, provided the practitioner avoid locations associated with the cervix and uterus, acupuncture is safe for both the mother and the fetus [64]. Despite the lack of evidence for the efficacy of acupuncture, the overall consensus is that acupuncture's benefits outweigh its risks, and that a trial of acupuncture can be considered in interested patients when the availability of other safe treatment options is limited.

6.3. Botulinum toxin

Botulinum toxin has been reported safe during the first trimester of pregnancy [65]. Although research for the use of Botox as a treatment for several chronic pain syndromes (e.g., myofascial pain, neuropathic pain) is promising, the only FDA-approved indications of Botox (serological types A and B) related to the treatment of chronic pain conditions are spasticity and chronic migraine. Evidence suggests that Botox is effective in providing pain relief for several months as a result of its long half-life [66]. Animal studies have shown some fetal damage, but the risk is uncertain in humans due to lack of sufficient evidence. Botox is classified by the FDA as a pregnancy category C drug. The current recommendation by the FDA is that Botox should be *"administered during pregnancy only if the potential benefits justifies the potential risk to the fetus."* In addition, other more conservative treatments should be exhausted first. If Botox is considered, the risk and benefits should be acknowledged by the patient prior to proceeding.

7. Interventions for pain management

7.1. Radiofrequency ablation

Radiofrequency ablation (RFA) is a process of nerve destruction via radiofrequency-generated heat by insertion of a catheter or electrode close to the target nerve under fluoroscopic guidance, confirming the correct location through sensory and motor testing, and applying a preset temperature for a fixed time period. This aims for neuromodulation of pain pathway by disruption of the transmission of nerve impulses from the pain generators to the central nervous system. The most common application of RFA is for the treatment of facet joint pain. Other applications include discogenic pain, radicular pain, and sacroiliac pain. Generally, a diagnostic and therapeutic block with local anesthetic with or without steroid is required to proceed with RFA. Current evidence suggests that RFA treatment has a modest, short-term benefit at best, with no long-term pain improvement, as supported by a recent meta-analysis

[67–69]. Contraindications to RFA are like those associated with other neuraxial procedures. Complications include increased pain, muscle spasms, numbness or paresthesias, infection, bleeding, superficial burns, damage to surrounding tissues, side effects of local anesthetics as well as fetal exposure to radiation. As a general rule, ultrasound and magnetic resonance imaging are the preferred imaging methods during pregnancy. Ionizing radiation (e.g., fluoroscopy) in large doses can have varying effects to the fetus via pregnancy loss, malformation, growth disturbances and mutagenic and carcinogenic effects depending on the stage of gestation. The most sensitive period of gestation to radiation occurs during organogenesis (weeks 2–8) [70]. The recommended maximum dose of radiation for the duration of pregnancy varies by source, but has been sighted as low as 500 mrem (or 0.5 Rads). For comparison, a pregnant interventional radiologist can expect an average dose of 30 mrem during a 40-week pregnancy if wearing double lead [71]. Radiation is not an absolute contraindication to RFA in the pregnant patient, and if clinically indicated RFA via fluoroscopy can be considered. Benefit–risk ratio of RFA is an important first step and if in doubt, a radiologist could be consulted. Since the average exposure of radiation during a fluoroscopic-guided RFA is not well defined in the literature, various methods should be employed to minimize the risk of exposure to the fetus. Some of these techniques include shielding the abdomen and pelvic region with lead, minimizing fluoroscopic exposure time, proper placement of the fluoroscope to maximize distance from the X-ray source, limit magnifications, narrowing of the fluoroscopic window (known as tight collimation) and proper gestational timing of the procedure [70]. Given the limited evidence of RFA, the lack of quality evidence of RFA during pregnancy, and the potential for radiation exposure to the fetus, RFAs should only be considered after failure of conservative treatments and an informed discussion with the patient.

7.2. Transcutaneous electrical nerve stimulation

Transcutaneous electrical nerve stimulation (TENS) is a technique of delivering low level of constant electrical impulses of variable frequencies, intensities and pulse waveforms to the epidermal surface with aim of inhibition of spinal cord interneurons and descending pain pathways [62, 72]. The indications for TENs are various, and examples include lower back pain and myofascial pain. Onset of pain relief takes on average 20–30 min in 75% of patients and 1 h in 95% of patients. The duration of pain relief varies among patients and conditions, but appears to be short term, decreasing over past several months of use [73]. During labor, TENS has demonstrated a benefit in acute pain relief, decreased analgesic use, and patient satisfaction [61, 74]. In contrast, two systemic analyses and a Cochrane review have not shown a significant reduction in pain [62, 75]. Technical errors from electrodes placement and timing could lead to interference with fetal heart monitoring and possible premature labor. All can easily be corrected by proper timing, proper anatomical placement of the devices, and removing the TENs if necessary [61]. Overall, the benefit of TENS for the treatment of chronic pain during pregnancy is not well studied in the literature. The general consensus is that the device's benefits outweigh its risks. TENS is easy to use and accessible over the counter. It provides a cost-effective, noninvasive, and potential pharmacologic sparing effect in pregnant patients and may be considered as an adjuvant for the safe treatment of chronic pain during pregnancy.

8. Special topics in pregnancy

8.1. Opioid use disorder in pregnancy

Opioid use during pregnancy has increased worldwide in recent years. In the United States, the prevalence of opioid abuse or dependence among pregnant women has increased from 1.7 per 1000 delivery admissions in 1998 to 3.9 per 1000 delivery admissions in 2011. The rate of unintended pregnancy has been reported as high as 86% in women with opioid use disorder, exposing the fetus right from conception [76]. Increase in opioid-related morbidity has been directly linked with the high prevalence of opioid prescription, which reaches 27–39% among pregnant women [77]. Opioid use disorder (OUD) is a pattern of opioid intake associated with significant clinical impairment and distress. OUD is diagnosed, as described in (**Table 4**) by the *Diagnostic and Statistical Manual of Mental Disorders, 5th Edition* (DSM-5), by at least **two** criteria within a **12-month** period [78].

Treatment of pregnant women with OUD has been shown to improve maternal and fetal outcome by decreasing the risk of relapse, maternal withdrawal symptoms, drug-seeking behaviors, and repeated cycles of intoxications [79, 80]. It also enhances the adherence to prenatal care. Opioid dependence in pregnancy is directly linked to placental insufficiency, fetal growth restriction, fetal death, abortions, premature delivery, preeclampsia, abruptio placentae, premature rupture of membranes, and postpartum hemorrhage. However, clear causality could not be established in the studied populations because of confounders in from of polydrug abuse, opioid withdrawal symptoms or coexisting maternal conditions [81]. Medical, nutritional, financial, psychological and socio-economical rampant in this patient population and should be taken into consideration when formulating a treatment plan.

Opioid use disorder (**OUD**)—DSM-5 Diagnosis by at least **2** criteria over **12** months.

- **Opioids intake** in larger amounts or over a longer period than was intended
- **Craving**, "strong desire or urge" to use opioids
- A persistent **desire** or unsuccessful efforts to cut down or control opioid use
- A great deal of **time** is spent to obtain, use or recover from the opioid
- **Failure** to fulfill **major role** obligations at work, school, or home
- **Recurrent opioid use** in physically hazardous situations
- **Reduction in important** social, or recreational activities.
- **Continued opioid** use despite the opioid related physical or psychological problem **Continued opioid** use despite the opioid related social or interpersonal problems
- **Tolerance**
- **Withdrawal**

Table 4. DSM-5 diagnostic criteria for OUD.

Methadone is still the standard treatment for the opioid dependence in many institutions due to its proven safety profile and established efficacy. Recently, the American College of Obstetrics and Gynecology (ACOG) has recommended buprenorphine as the first line therapy in OUD [82]. The interest is growing for buprenorphine after retrospective reports for its benefit of lower rates, lesser severity of NAS, lower morphine doses used for NAS, and a shorter stay in NICU [83]. Buprenorphine has a ceiling effect with expected low risk for overdose compared with methadone. The efficacy of buprenorphine as a substitution therapy has been debated because it was found that the patients on buprenorphine have less compliance rate and more reversion to other opioid drug abuse; however, those reports were biased and have different patient characteristics [34]. Both buprenorphine and methadone are considered safe with no significant harm and have shown good outcomes in OUD treatment [35].

8.2. Neonatal abstinence syndrome

As a shadow of opioid crisis and high prevalence of maternal opioid exposure, the incidence of NAS has increased worldwide. In the USA, a 400% increase in the incidence of NAS were reported and 5.8 up to 30 per 1000 hospital births in 2012, compared with 1.2 in 2000 [84, 85]. In 2012, one NAS-affected infant was born every 25 min in the United States [85].

Neonatal abstinence syndrome (NAS) is a neonatal drug withdrawal syndrome that occurs after opioids exposure in utero. The opioid is the main culprit for the withdrawal; however, other substances have also been reported, including alcohol, benzodiazepines, nicotine, and psychiatric medications such as antidepressants or antipsychotics [86]. The source of the opioid could be from clinician-approved use of prescription opioids for pain relief, or abuse of prescription opioids or illicit use (e.g., heroin); or medication-assisted treatment (MAT) of opioid use disorder.

In utero, fetal exposure to opioids during pregnancy is associated with a 60–80% risk of NAS [87]. However, the onset and severity are multifactorial and variable. They depend on gestational age, birth weight, maternal opioid dosage, concomitant use of other psychoactive medications and pharmacogenomics. NAS usually manifests within 2–3 days after birth with clinical signs of withdrawal as summarized in **Table 5** [88].

Multiple brain volumetric studies have reported a small volume of cortex, deep midbrain, brainstem, and thin cerebellar cortex in infants with in utero polydrug exposure including opiates [86].

Autonomic nervous system activation	**Central nervous system irritability**
Fever—sweating	High-pitched continuous crying
Temperature dysregulation	Irritability—decreased sleep
Increased respiratory rate	Tremors—muscle hypertonicity
Nasal stuffiness, sneezing	Seizures
Gastrointestinal dysfunction	**Cardiovascular dysfunction**
Feeding difficulties	Tachycardia—hypertension
Vomiting—loose diarrhea	Hypotension in case of collapse

Table 5. Summary of neonatal abstinence syndrome (NAS).

Long-term neurodevelopmental sequelae such as attention deficit disorders (ADD) and disruptive behavior have been reported in NAS. Therefore, long-term psychiatric follow-up is warranted [89]. Inpatient monitoring for 4–7 days for neonates with known in utero exposure to opioids is recommended by the American Association of Pediatrics (AAP) [88].

Non-pharmacological management is the initial approach for NAS. It entails keeping the neonate in calm, soothing environment with minimal stimulation, repeated maternal contact, and frequent hypercaloric meals [90]. Pharmacologic treatment is usually needed. This constitutes oral morphine as the first line agent and either clonidine or phenobarbital as the second line agent [85]. Once withdrawal symptoms are stable for 48 h, pharmacological weaning can be started. Breastfeeding is recommended in general even for mothers on methadone or buprenorphine treatment, as long as no other contraindications are present (e.g., HIV, illicit drug use) [82].

9. Recommendations summary

Chronic pain management in pregnancy is challenging. A multidisciplinary team approach and multimodal pain protocols are highly recommended. Optimum management includes a detailed review of the patient's comorbidities and considerations for behavioral and other socioeconomic factors that could affect chronic pain conditions. The safest approach is by following a goal-directed strategy that minimizes or optimizes opioid usage. Opioid sparing strategies include early alternative pain therapies such as exercise, physical therapy, behavioral changes, and non-opioid analgesics. Lifestyle and behavioral changes start with open, effective, and compassionate communication with the patient. The initial and follow-up visits should include patient education on different pharmacological options and alternative non-pharmacological modalities. Patients should be encouraged to take an active role in their own treatment plan. Acetaminophen is usually the first line drug for mild to moderate pain in any stage of pregnancy. Although ibuprofen is the non-steroidal anti-inflammatory drug (NSAID) of choice, it is contraindicated after 28 weeks of gestation as it could cause premature closure of the ductus arteriosus and impair fetal kidney function. Only in severe acute musculoskeletal pain, opioids should be used. Caution should be taken as peripartum administration is associated with neonatal respiratory depression. Additionally, a long-term therapy, particularly in late pregnancy, is associated with adaptation disorders and neonatal withdrawal symptoms. Once the opioids are indicated in a reproductive age woman, the benefits and risks of opioid use should be discussed. However, concerns about NAS or opioid abuse should not be a barrier for optimal pain management in pregnancy as long as a cautious and balanced approach is followed. Opioid prescriptions should be initiated with a drug monitoring program that could help to identify opioid use disorder or drug misuse. Concurrent opioid and benzodiazepines use should be avoided whenever possible. Opioid overdose is associated with high maternal and fetal mortality and morbidity. In case of overdose, substance abuse disorder, or higher opioid dosages (≥50 MME/day), naloxone should be prescribed. To avoid relapse, which is associated with very high morbidity in pregnant women with opioid use disorder, an opioid agonist (buprenorphine or methadone) is the recommended first line therapy in combination with behavioral therapy. Antiepileptic drugs are contraindicated during pregnancy as they carry a teratogenic risk; however, well-studied antidepressants, such as sertraline and amitriptyline can be used for chronic pain with the appropriate indications. Sumatriptan is safe to use in pregnant patients with migraine.

Acknowledgements

Special thanks for Dr. Raval Chetankumar, assistant professor of Clinical Anesthesiology at Weill Cornell University, Qatar and Dr. Brahim Boudjenah, senior anesthesia specialist in Hamad Medical Corporation, Qatar for their valuable comments, chapter editing, and reviewing. The publication of this article was funded by the Qatar National Library.

Author details

Ahmed Zaghw[1]*, Mohamed Koronfel[2], Edward Podgorski[3], Sara Siddiqui[1], Arif Valliani[1], Arunabha Karmakar[1] and Jaffar Khan[1]

*Address all correspondence to: azaghw@hamad.qa

1 Hamad General Hospital, Weill Cornell University, Doha, Qatar

2 Cleveland Clinic, Cleveland, Ohio, USA

3 Jackson Memorial Hospital, University of Miami, Miami, Florida, USA

References

[1] Elden H, Gutke A, Kjellby-Wendt G, Fagevik-Olsen M, Ostgaard H-C. Predictors and consequences of long-term pregnancy-related pelvic girdle pain: A longitudinal follow-up study. BMC Musculoskeletal Disorders. 2016 Dec 12;**17**(1):276

[2] Martin CE, Longinaker N, Terplan M. Recent trends in treatment admissions for prescription opioid abuse during pregnancy. Journal of Substance Abuse Treatment. 2015 Jan;**48**(1):37-42

[3] Kristiansson P, Svardsudd K, von Schoultz B. Back pain during pregnancy: A prospective study. Spine (Phila Pa 1976). 1996 Mar;**21**(6):702-709

[4] Ritchie JR. Orthopedic considerations during pregnancy. Clinical Obstetrics and Gynecology. 2003 Jun;**46**(2):456-466

[5] Kovacs FM, Garcia E, Royuela A, Gonzalez L, Abraira V. Prevalence and factors associated with low back pain and pelvic girdle pain during pregnancy: A multicenter study conducted in the Spanish National Health Service. Spine (Phila Pa 1976). 2012 Aug;**37**(17):1516-1533

[6] To WW, Wong MW. Persistence of back pain symptoms after pregnancy and bone mineral density changes as measured by quantitative ultrasound—A two year longitudinal follow up study. BMC Musculoskeletal Disorders. 2011 Feb;**12**:55

[7] Marshall SA, Ng L, Unemori EN, Girling JE, Parry LJ. Relaxin deficiency results in increased expression of angiogenesis- and remodelling-related genes in the uterus of early pregnant mice but does not affect endometrial angiogenesis prior to implantation. Reproductive Biology and Endocrinology. 2016 Mar 22;**14**(1):11

[8] Soh YM, Tiwari A, Mahendroo M, Conrad KP, Parry LJ. Relaxin regulates hyaluronan synthesis and aquaporins in the cervix of late pregnant mice. Endocrinology. 2012 Dec;**153**(12):6054-6064

[9] Heenan AP, Wolfe LA, Davies GAL, McGrath MJ. Effects of human pregnancy on fluid regulation responses to short-term exercise. Journal of Applied Physiology. 2003 Dec;**95**(6):2321-2327

[10] McMahon SB, Dmitrieva N, Koltzenburg M. Visceral pain. British Journal of Anaesthesia. 1995 Aug;**75**(2):132-144

[11] Tripp DA, Nickel JC, Fitzgerald MP, Mayer R, Stechyson N, Hsieh A. Sexual functioning, catastrophizing, depression, and pain, as predictors of quality of life in women with interstitial cystitis/painful bladder syndrome. Urology. 2009 May;**73**(5):987-992

[12] Scriven MW, Jones DA, McKnight L. Current concepts review. Musculoskeletal considerations in pregnancy. The Journal of Bone and Joint Surgery. American Volume. 1995 Sep;**77**(9):1465

[13] Eshed I, Miloh-Raz H, Dulitzki M, Lidar Z, Aharoni D, Liberman B, et al. Peripartum changes of the sacroiliac joints on MRI: Increasing mechanical load correlating with signs of edema and inflammation kindling spondyloarthropathy in the genetically prone. Clinical Rheumatology. 2015 Aug 26;**34**(8):1419-1426

[14] Hughes SE, Spelman T, Gray OM, Boz C, Trojano M, Lugaresi A, et al. Predictors and dynamics of postpartum relapses in women with multiple sclerosis. Multiple Sclerosis. 2014 May 9;**20**(6):739-746

[15] Zrour SH, Boumiza R, Sakly N, Mannai R, Korbaa W, Younes M, et al. The impact of pregnancy on rheumatoid arthritis outcome: The role of maternofetal HLA class II disparity. Joint, Bone, Spine. 2010 Jan;**77**(1):36-40

[16] May S, Littlewood C, Bishop A. Reliability of procedures used in the physical examination of non-specific low back pain: A systematic review. The Australian Journal of Physiotherapy. 2006;**52**(2):91-102

[17] Petersen T, Laslett M, Juhl C. Clinical classification in low back pain: Best-evidence diagnostic rules based on systematic reviews. BMC Musculoskeletal Disorders. 2017 Dec 12;**18**(1):188

[18] Chou R, Fu R, Carrino JA, Deyo RA. Imaging strategies for low-back pain: Systematic review and meta-analysis. Lancet (London, England). 2009 Feb 7;**373**(9662):463-472

[19] Vleeming A, Albert HB, Ostgaard HC, Sturesson B, Stuge B. European guidelines for the diagnosis and treatment of pelvic girdle pain. European Spine Journal. 2008 Jun 8;**17**(6):794-819

[20] Adams SM, Blanco C, Chaudhry HJ, et al. First do no harm: Marshaling Clinician Leadership to Counter the Opioid Epidemic. Washington, DC: National Academy of Medicine; 2017

[21] Evers S, Afra J, Frese A, Goadsby PJ, Linde M, May A, et al. EFNS guideline on the drug treatment of migraine-revised report of an EFNS task force. European Journal of Neurology. 2009 Sep;**16**(9):968-981

[22] Amundsen S, Nordeng H, Nezvalová-Henriksen K, Stovner LJ, Spigset O. Pharmacological treatment of migraine during pregnancy and breastfeeding. Nature Reviews. Neurology. 2015;**11**(4):209-219

[23] Cassina M, Di Gianantonio E, Toldo I, Battistella PA, Clementi M. Migraine therapy during pregnancy and lactation. Expert Opinion on Drug Safety. 2010 Nov 27;**9**(6):937-948

[24] Padua L, Di PA, Pazzaglia C, Liotta GA, Librante A, Mondelli M. Systematic review of pregnancy-related carpal tunnel syndrome. Muscle & Nerve. 2010 Nov;**42**(5):697-702

[25] Turgut F, Cetinşahinahin M, Turgut M, Bölükbaşi O. The management of carpal tunnel syndrome in pregnancy. Journal of Clinical Neuroscience. 2001 Jul;**8**(4):332-334

[26] Roditi D, Robinson ME. The role of psychological interventions in the management of patients with chronic pain. Psychology Research and Behavior Management. 2011;**4**:41-49

[27] Hanna MN, González-Fernández M, Barrett AD, Williams KA, Pronovost P. Does patient perception of pain control affect patient satisfaction across surgical units in a tertiary teaching hospital? American Journal of Medical Quality. 2012 Sep 16;**27**(5):411-416

[28] Vallerand AH, Templin T, Hasenau SM, Riley-Doucet C. Factors that affect functional status in patients with cancer-related pain. Pain. 2007 Nov;**132**(1-2):82-90

[29] Arnstein P, Caudill M, Mandle CL, Norris A, Beasley R. Self efficacy as a mediator of the relationship between pain intensity, disability and depression in chronic pain patients. Pain. 1999 Apr;**80**(3):483-491

[30] Stuge B, Hilde G, Vøllestad N. Physical therapy for pregnancy-related low back and pelvic pain: A systematic review. Acta Obstetricia et Gynecologica Scandinavica. 2003 Nov;**82**(11):983-990

[31] Brent RL. Environmental causes of human congenital malformations: The pediatrician's role in dealing with these complex clinical problems caused by a multiplicity of environmental and genetic factors. Pediatrics. 2004 Apr;**113**(4 Suppl):957-968

[32] U.S. Food and Drug Administration. Labeling – Pregnancy and Lactation Labeling (Drugs) Final Rule. 2014. Available from: https://www.fda.gov/Drugs/DevelopmentApprovalProcess/DevelopmentResources/Labeling/ucm093307.htm [Accessed: 2018-06-29]

[33] Desai RJ, Hernandez-Diaz S, Bateman BT, Huybrechts KF. Increase in prescription opioid use during pregnancy among medicaid-enrolled women. Obstetrics and Gynecology. 2014 May;**123**(5):997-1002

[34] Mattick RP, Kimber J, Breen C, Davoli M. Buprenorphine maintenance versus placebo or methadone maintenance for opioid dependence. Mattick RP, Editor. The Cochrane Database Systematic Reviews. 2008 Apr 16;**2**:CD002207

[35] Brogly SB, Saia KA, Walley AY, Du HM, Sebastiani P. Prenatal buprenorphine versus methadone exposure and neonatal outcomes: Systematic review and meta-analysis. American Journal of Epidemiology. 2014 Oct 1;**180**(7):673-686

[36] U.S. Food and Drug Administration. FDA has reviewed possible risks of pain medicine use during pregnancy. 2015. Available from: https://www.fda.gov/Drugs/DrugSafety/ucm429117.htm [Accessed: 2018-06-29]

[37] Niesters M, Overdyk F, Smith T, Aarts L, Dahan A. Opioid-induced respiratory depression in paediatrics: A review of case reports. British Journal of Anaesthesia. 2013 Feb; **110**(2):175-182

[38] Werler MM, Mitchell AA, Hernandez-Diaz S, Honein MA. Use of over-the-counter medications during pregnancy. American Journal of Obstetrics and Gynecology. 2005 Sep;**193**(3 Pt 1):771-777

[39] Rebordosa C, Kogevinas M, Horváth-Puhó E, Nørgård B, Morales M, Czeizel AE, et al. Acetaminophen use during pregnancy: Effects on risk for congenital abnormalities. American Journal of Obstetrics and Gynecology. 2008 Feb;**198**(2):178.e1-178.e7

[40] Cooper M, Langley K, Thapar A. Antenatal acetaminophen use and attention-deficit/hyperactivity disorder: An interesting observed association but too early to infer causality. JAMA Pediatrics. 2014 Apr 1;**168**(4):306-307

[41] Kaandorp SP, Goddijn M, van der Post JAM, Hutten BA, Verhoeve HR, Hamulyák K, et al. Aspirin plus heparin or aspirin alone in women with recurrent miscarriage. The New England Journal of Medicine. 2010 Apr 29;**362**(17):1586-1596

[42] Schulz P, Steimer T. Psychotropic medication, psychiatric disorders, and higher brain functions. Dialogues in Clinical Neuroscience. 2000 Sep;**2**(3):177-182

[43] Antenatal and Postnatal Mental Health: Clinical Management and Service Guidance; Clinical Guideline; 2014. Available from: http://nice.org.uk/guidance/cg192

[44] Grigoriadis S, VonderPorten EH, Mamisashvili L, Roerecke M, Rehm J, Dennis C-L, et al. Antidepressant exposure during pregnancy and congenital malformations: Is there an association? A systematic review and meta-analysis of the best evidence. The Journal of Clinical Psychiatry. 2013 Apr 15;**74**(4):e293-e308

[45] Einarson A. Antidepressants and pregnancy: Complexities of producing evidence-based information. CMAJ. 2010 Jul 13;**182**(10):1017-1018

[46] Marcus SM, Heringhausen JE. Depression in childbearing women: When depression complicates pregnancy. Primary Care. 2009 Mar;**36**(1):151-165. ix

[47] Gentile S. Tricyclic antidepressants in pregnancy and puerperium. Expert Opinion on Drug Safety. 2014 Feb 3;**13**(2):207-225

[48] National Collaborating Centre for Mental Health (UK). Antenatal and Postnatal Mental Health: Clinical Management and Service Guidance: NICE Clinical Guidelines: Updated Edition. Leicester (UK): British Psychological Society; No. 192. 2014

[49] Meador KJ, Pennell PB, Harden CL, Gordon JC, Tomson T, Kaplan PW, et al. Pregnancy registries in epilepsy: A consensus statement on health outcomes. Neurology. 2008 Sep 30;**71**(14):1109-1117

[50] Tomson T, Battino D, Bonizzoni E, Craig J, Lindhout D, Sabers A, et al. Dose-dependent risk of malformations with antiepileptic drugs: An analysis of data from the EURAP epilepsy and pregnancy registry. Lancet Neurology. 2011 Jul;**10**(7):609-617

[51] Patorno E, Bateman BT, Huybrechts KF, MacDonald SC, Cohen JM, Desai RJ, et al. Pregabalin use early in pregnancy and the risk of major congenital malformations. Neurology. 2017 May 23;**88**(21):2020-2025

[52] Brunner E, Falk DM, Jones M, Dey DK, Shatapathy CC. Olanzapine in pregnancy and breastfeeding: A review of data from global safety surveillance. BMC Pharmacology and Toxicology. 2013 Aug 1;**14**(1):38

[53] Geneen LJ, Moore RA, Clarke C, Martin D, Colvin LA, Smith BH. Physical activity and exercise for chronic pain in adults: An overview of cochrane reviews. Cochrane Database of Systematic Reviews. 2017 Apr 24;**4**:CD011279

[54] Stagg NJ, Mata HP, Ibrahim MM, Henriksen EJ, Porreca F, Vanderah TW, et al. Regular exercise reverses sensory hypersensitivity in a rat neuropathic pain model: Role of endogenous opioids. Anesthesiology. 2011 Apr;**114**(4):940-948

[55] Messier SP, Mihalko SL, Legault C, Miller GD, Nicklas BJ, DeVita P, et al. Effects of intensive diet and exercise on knee joint loads, inflammation, and clinical outcomes among overweight and obese adults with knee osteoarthritis: The IDEA randomized clinical trial. Journal of the American Medical Association. 2013 Sep 25;**310**(12):1263-1273

[56] Fletcher GF, Ades PA, Kligfield P, Arena R, Balady GJ, Bittner VA, et al. Exercise standards for testing and training: A scientific statement from the American Heart Association. Circulation. 2013 Aug 20;**128**(8):873-934

[57] Thompson PD, Franklin BA, Balady GJ, Blair SN, Corrado D, Estes NAM, et al. Exercise and acute cardiovascular events placing the risks into perspective: A scientific statement from the American Heart Association Council on Nutrition, Physical Activity, and Metabolism and the Council on Clinical Cardiology. Circulation. 2007 May 1;**115**(17):2358-2368

[58] Stuge B, Laerum E, Kirkesola G, Vøllestad N. The efficacy of a treatment program focusing on specific stabilizing exercises for pelvic girdle pain after pregnancy: A randomized controlled trial. Spine (Phila Pa 1976). 2004 Feb 15;**29**(4):351-359

[59] Carlsson C. Acupuncture mechanisms for clinically relevant long-term effects–reconsideration and a hypothesis. Acupuncture in Medicine. 2002 Aug;**20**(2-3):82-99

[60] Nesheim B-I, Kinge R, Berg B, Alfredsson B, Allgot E, Hove G, et al. Acupuncture during labor can reduce the use of meperidine: A controlled clinical study. The Clinical Journal of Pain;**19**(3):187-191

[61] Simkin P, Bolding A. Update on nonpharmacologic approaches to relieve labor pain and prevent suffering. Journal of Midwifery & Women's Health;**49**(6):489-504

[62] Liddle SD, Pennick V. Interventions for preventing and treating low-back and pelvic pain during pregnancy. Cochrane Database of Systematic Reviews. 2015 Sep 30;**9**:CD001139

[63] Linde K, Allais G, Brinkhaus B, Manheimer E, Vickers A, White AR. Acupuncture for tension-type headache. Linde K, Editor. Cochrane Database of Systematic Reviews. 2009 Jan 21;**1**:CD007587

[64] Melchart D, Weidenhammer W, Streng A, Reitmayr S, Hoppe A, Ernst E, et al. Prospective investigation of adverse effects of acupuncture in 97,733 patients. Archives of Internal Medicine. 2004 Jan 12;**164**(1):104-105

[65] Oh H-M, Chung ME. Botulinum toxin for neuropathic pain: A review of the literature. Toxins (Basel). 2015 Aug 14;**7**(8):3127-3154

[66] Patil S, Willett O, Thompkins T, Hermann R, Ramanathan S, Cornett EM, et al. Botulinum toxin: Pharmacology and therapeutic roles in pain states. Current Pain and Headache Reports. 2016 Mar 15;**20**(3):15

[67] van Wijk RMAW, Geurts JWM, Wynne HJ, Hammink E, Buskens E, Lousberg R, et al. Radiofrequency denervation of lumbar facet joints in the treatment of chronic low back pain: A randomized, double-blind, sham lesion-controlled trial. The Clinical Journal of Pain;**21**(4):335-344

[68] Cohen SP, Hurley RW, Buckenmaier CC, Kurihara C, Morlando B, Dragovich A. Randomized placebo-controlled study evaluating lateral branch radiofrequency denervation for sacroiliac joint pain. Anesthesiology. 2008 Aug;**109**(2):279-288

[69] Bogduk N. Lumbar radiofrequency neurotomy. The Clinical Journal of Pain. 2006 May;**22**(4):409

[70] Vu CT, Elder DH. Pregnancy and the working interventional radiologist. Seminars in Interventional Radiology. 2013 Dec 20;**30**(4):403-407

[71] Leggett LE, Soril LJJ, Lorenzetti DL, Noseworthy T, Steadman R, Tiwana S, et al. Radiofrequency ablation for chronic low back pain: A systematic review of randomized controlled trials. Pain Research & Management;**19**(5):e146-e153

[72] Sluka KA, Walsh D. Transcutaneous electrical nerve stimulation: Basic science mechanisms and clinical effectiveness. The Journal of Pain. 2003 Apr;**4**(3):109-121

[73] Johnson MI, Ashton CH, Thompson JW. An in-depth study of long-term users of transcutaneous electrical nerve stimulation (TENS). Implications for clinical use of TENS. Pain. 1991 Mar;**44**(3):221-229

[74] Chao A-S, Chao A, Wang T-H, Chang Y-C, Peng H-H, Chang S-D, et al. Pain relief by applying transcutaneous electrical nerve stimulation (TENS) on acupuncture points during the first stage of labor: A randomized double-blind placebo-controlled trial. Pain. 2007 Feb;**127**(3):214-220

[75] Carroll D, Tramèr M, McQuay H, Nye B, Moore A. Transcutaneous electrical nerve stimulation in labour pain: A systematic review. British Journal of Obstetrics and Gynaecology. 1997 Feb;**104**(2):169-175

[76] Heil SH, Jones HE, Arria A, Kaltenbach K, Coyle M, Fischer G, et al. Unintended pregnancy in opioid-abusing women. Journal of Substance Abuse Treatment. 2011 Mar;**40**(2):199-202

[77] Ailes EC, Dawson AL, Lind JN, Gilboa SM, Frey MT, Broussard CS, et al. Opioid prescription claims among women of reproductive age—United States, 2008-2012. MMWR. Morbidity and Mortality Weekly Report. 2015 Jan;**64**(2):37-41

[78] American Psychiatric Association. Diagnostic and Statistical Manual of Mental Disorders. Fifth edition, American Psychiatric Association; 2013. DOI: 10.1176/appi.books.9780890425596

[79] WHO. Guidelines for Identification and Management of Substance Use and Substance Use Disorders in Pregnancy. Geneva, Switzerland: WHO Press, World Health Organization; 2014. ISBN: 9789241548731. Available from: http://apps.who.int/iris/bitstream/handle/10665/107130/9789241548731_eng.pdf;jsessionid=1778A5AE016CB48996021D538AF83F87?sequence=1

[80] Young JL, Martin PR. Treatment of opioid dependence in the setting of pregnancy. The Psychiatric Clinics of North America. 2012 Jun;**35**(2):441-460

[81] Maeda A, Bateman BT, Clancy CR, Creanga AA, Leffert LR. Opioid abuse and dependence during pregnancy: Temporal trends and obstetrical outcomes. Anesthesiology. 2014 Dec;**121**(6):1158-1165

[82] ACOG Committee on Health Care for Underserved Women, American Society of Addiction Medicine. ACOG Committee Opinion No. 524: Opioid abuse, dependence, and addiction in pregnancy. Obstetrics and Gynecology. 2012 May;**119**(5):1070-1076

[83] Zedler BK, Mann AL, Kim MM, Amick HR, Joyce AR, Murrelle EL, et al. Buprenorphine compared with methadone to treat pregnant women with opioid use disorder: a systematic review and meta-analysis of safety in the mother, fetus and child. Addiction. Dec 2016;**111**(12):2115-2128

[84] Patrick SW, Davis MM, Lehmann CU, Lehman CU, Cooper WO. Increasing incidence and geographic distribution of neonatal abstinence syndrome: United States 2009-2012. Journal of Perinatology. 2015 Aug 30;**35**(8):650-655

[85] Kocherlakota P. Neonatal abstinence syndrome. Pediatrics. 2014 Aug 1;**134**(2):e547-e561

[86] Walhovd KB, Moe V, Slinning K, Due-Tønnessen P, Bjørnerud A, Dale AM, et al. Volumetric cerebral characteristics of children exposed to opiates and other substances in utero. NeuroImage. 2007 Jul 15;**36**(4):1331-1344

[87] Doberczak TM, Kandall SR, Wilets I. Neonatal opiate abstinence syndrome in term and preterm infants. The Journal of Pediatrics. 1991 Jun;**118**(6):933-937

[88] Hudak ML, Tan RC, Committee on Drugs, Committee on Fetus and Newborn, American Academy of Pediatrics. Neonatal drug withdrawal. Pediatrics. 2012 Feb 1;**129**(2):e540-e560

[89] Ornoy A. The impact of intrauterine exposure versus postnatal environment in neurodevelopmental toxicity: Long-term neurobehavioral studies in children at risk for developmental disorders. Toxicology Letters. 2003 Apr 11;**140-141**:171-181

[90] Jansson LM, Velez M, Harrow C. The opioid-exposed newborn: Assessment and pharmacologic management. Journal of Opioid Management;**5**(1):47-55

Chapter 6

Pain Management in Patients with Impaired Kidney Function

Shakhsanam Mirishova and
Yasser Mahmoud Hammad Ali Hammad

Additional information is available at the end of the chapter

http://dx.doi.org/10.5772/intechopen.81695

Abstract

Huge numbers of patients referred to pain service have kidney function impairment to some extent. Pain physicians face puzzling cases and may find themselves struggling and divided between the decisions of providing adequate pain reliever, at the same time avoiding further damage to kidneys, and excessive accumulation of medications and their metabolites, also negative interactions with patient's other medications. In this chapter, we will reason about the prevalence of pain in patients with renal impairment, pharmacodynamics and pharmacokinetics of pain medications in this group, optimization of pain control, preferred choice of drugs according to the level of kidney damage, and feasibility of alternative pain management techniques.

Keywords: impaired kidney function (IKF), chronic kidney disease (CKD), acute pain, chronic pain

1. Introduction

Across all subspecialties, pain is the most encountered problem. It is particularly difficult to deal with in patients with organ dysfunction such as acute or chronic kidney failure, due to the fact that most medications depend on kidneys for clearance. Moreover, pharmacokinetics becomes almost unpredictable due to fluctuations in kidney function depending on patient factors such as volume status, other medication actions, or enzyme build of certain individual.

2. Epidemiology

The prevalence of pain in patients with chronic kidney disease (CKD) has been shown in many epidemiologic studies, and all of them unanimously demonstrate that pain is more common in CKD patients than the general population.

Murtagh et al., in a cross-sectional survey of symptoms prevalence in stage 5 chronic kidney disease managed without dialysis, found that pain was present in 53% (42–63%) of total 66 patients with a mean age of 82 ± 6.6 years [1].

Davison et al. have analyzed publications from 1992 to 2009 and concluded that 58% of CKD patients are suffering from pain, 49% of those patients rated their pain as moderate to severe [2].

As quality of life is greatly diminished by any kind of pain, it has been studied in CKD patients as part of symptom burden, for example [3], older patients found musculoskeletal symptoms, including pain in bones/joints (69% of 283 CKD Stage 1–5 patients), are more disturbing and bothersome, while younger patients found that reduced concentration is more intrusive. Perlman et al. also demonstrated that the presence of pain was associated with lower quality-of-life scores in a multicenter cross-sectional analysis of 634 patients with CKD [4].

Additionally, in prospective cohort study of 205 Canadian hemodialysis (HD) patients, 50% of them reported pain which was related to those who was on longer HD therapy, 52.5 months with pain versus 37.7 months for those without pain.

The etiology of pain was multiple in 18.4% of patients with pain, among which musculoskeletal was the most frequent (50.5%); same study found that almost one third of all patients with pain were not on any painkillers, and authors concluded that pain management was ineffective in 74.8 of patients [5].

Pain in CKD patients is an important factor, which immensely affects quality of life. Weisbord et al. showed clear correlation between symptom excess and severity with diminished quality of life. If they had considered pain-related symptoms such as muscle cramps, headache, and chest pain in pain group, the prevalence would have increased to 50–85% [6].

Moreover, CKD patients with pain tend to decide to withdraw from HD more often; as shown by Davison and Jhangri, they also were more depressed and suffered sleep disturbances [7].

3. Definition and staging of chronic kidney disease

It is very important to identify the degree of IKF and the nature of CKD and on what stage it is, because these factors will guide the management of pain and to some extent predict pain medication pharmacokinetics.

Definition for CKD must have the following criteria:

http://dx.doi.org/10.5772/intechopen.81695

1. Kidney damage for 3 months or more, represented by structural or functional abnormalities of the kidney, with or without decreased GFR and manifested by following:
   a. Pathological abnormalities
   b. Markers of kidney damage, such as abnormalities in the composition of the blood or urine, or abnormalities in imaging tests
2. GFR less than 60 mL/min/1.73 m^2 for more than 3 months with or without kidney damage [8]

Evaluation of kidney function is more dependent on GFR or the presence of other markers of kidney damage rather than a single serum creatinine reading.

Stages of CKD according to GFR are described in **Table 1**.

Stages	GFR (mL/min/1.73 m^2)	Terms/uremic symptoms
Stage 1	90 or more	Normal function/asymptomatic
Stage 2	60–89	Mild/asymptomatic
Stage 3	30–59	Moderate/mild symptoms
Stage 4	15–29	Severe/mild to moderate symptoms
Stage 5	15 or less	End-stage renal disease/moderate to severe symptoms, may require dialysis

Table 1. Stages of chronic kidney disease according to glomerular filtration rate [8].

4. Pain in patients with CKD

4.1. Acute pain in patients with CKD

The cause for acute pain is mainly acute injury such as surgery, procedures, and childbirth. It can be caused by acute inflammation or ischemia as well, for example, acute abdomen, colic, and ischemic heart diseases. Treatment should be directed to reduce the pain as soon as possible with multiple modalities; at the same time, the primary cause should be addressed.

Blocking the pain along different parts of pain pathway allows reducing the required doses and diminishing side effects. This approach has been defined as multimodal analgesia.

Multimodal analgesia can be achieved by combining systemic paracetamol, NSAID, opioids, and local anesthetics according to patient's condition. All these medications may require dose adjustment, and locoregional anesthesia may raise a concern of hematoma formation due to reduced platelet activity and anticoagulant use in patients receiving hemodialysis [9].

Choice and dosage of medications depend on the condition of the kidneys; here the staging can roughly guide physicians to correct regimen.

For example, in stages 1 and 2, kidney function is preserved well enough to excrete the medications and their metabolites. But still, kidney function tests should be frequently done so not to miss any deterioration due to trauma, dehydration, and surgical stress during perioperative period. In young patients who are not taking other nephrotoxic medications and in stage 1, acetaminophen plus short course of NSAIDs could be used. NSAIDs should not be used in stage 2 with GFR 60–89 mL/min/1.73 m^2. Locoregional anesthesia must be used when applicable, especially for postoperative pain and trauma patients. In cases of moderate to severe pain, opioids should be added including tramadol, with or without gabapentinoids (Gabapentin or Pregabalin) to supplement for neuropathic pain, especially in trauma [9].

In stages 3 and 4, kidney function significantly reduced (GFR between 15 and 59 mL/min/1.73 m^2) which mandate all the pain medications to be dose adjusted and NSAIDs to be avoided. Acetaminophen should be used in regular doses for mild pain, reduced dose tramadol may be added, and for stronger pain, opioid such as fentanyl or hydromorphone may be useful. Morphine and codeine are not recommended. Regional anesthesia proves to be a valuable modality to avoid opioids and their undesired properties, especially in this stage, but should be avoided in individuals with impaired platelet function and/or coagulation. Reduced doses of gabapentinoids are considered in neuropathic pain, and caution should be taken when patients receive concomitant opioids. A decrease in around 50% of the dose for each 50% decline in GFR or CCr and an increase in the time interval between the doses are recommended [9, 10].

Acute pain management in end-stage renal disease (ESRD) patients follows the same above-mentioned principles; in addition to it, more than half of them may already have been experiencing chronic pain as well. Moreover, these patients are usually malnourished and have many other multiple concomitant diseases. If they are already undergoing dialysis, sudden drop in serum concentration of pain medications and exacerbation of pain is expected. Acetaminophen may be used in regular doses of 4 g/day, but general condition of patient and other organ system diseases may require dose reduction. NSAIDs should be avoided in ESRD; even if nephrotoxicity is not of a concern, they cause gastrointestinal damage, electrolyte disturbances, and hypertension. Cyclo-oxygenase-2 inhibitors are also considered unsafe as they contribute to already existent multiple risk factors for myocardial ischemia in this group of patients [11].

Morphine, codeine, and meperidine produce active metabolites, in which clearance depends on kidney function. In ESRD patients, the accumulation of active metabolites of opioids produces excessive somnolence, as well as more dangerous complications such as respiratory depression, seizures, myoclonus, and exacerbation of acidosis. Safe alternative to these long-acting opioids are fentanyl, alfentanil, and adjusted dose of hydromorphone [12]. These can be best given as PCA in acute pain cases if strong opioids are required.

4.2. Chronic pain in CKD patients

Chronic pain is defined by Treede et al. as pain that persists past normal healing time [13] and hence lacks the acute warning function of physiological nociception [14]. It may be due to prolonged tissue injury with persistent activation of nociceptors or other undefined mechanisms [15].

Recommendations of the WHO for cancer pain and its three-step approach can be tailored to manage pharmacologic treatment of chronic pain in CKD patients [2, 15, 16]. In patients with mild pain, acetaminophen may suffice, and if NSAIDs are required, care should be taken to avoid other medications which worsen the hemodynamics (compounds that affect the renin-angiotensin-aldosterone system). NSAIDs should be avoided in patients with impaired cardiac output or with dehydration.

For moderate pain, weak opioid tramadol may be added, but codeine and dihydrocodeine should not be prescribed. Tramadol dose is adjusted according to CKD stage, given in regular doses for stages 1 and 2, but is reduced by 50% in advanced stages of CKD.

Severe pain requires the use of strong opioids, preferably those without active metabolites such as methadone, fentanyl, and oxycodone. Although, oxycodone is mainly metabolized in the liver, around 20% is eliminated by kidneys. For that reason, it may be wise to reduce the dose according to CKD stage; in mild renal failure, up to 50% of normal dose should be given, and in advanced stages, 25% of normal dose and increase in dosing interval should be done. In patients with consistent pain, fentanyl patch can be a good option [15, 16].

In all steps of WHO ladder, adjuvant medications should be added and tailored to a particular type of pain. If patient is experiencing neuropathic pain, antidepressants and anticonvulsants should be added to pain regimen. Musculoskeletal pain may have spastic component; thus muscle relaxants are beneficial. Bisphosphonates are considered adjuvant for bone pain due to malignancy. There is at least one meta-analysis to support the effect of omega-3 polyunsaturated fatty acids as an effective adjunct for joint pain (rheumatoid arthritis, inflammatory bowel disease) [17].

Pharmacologic treatment of chronic neuropathic pain for adults should be done in a stepwise approach. The first line is tricyclic antidepressants (TCAs), followed by selective serotonin norepinephrine reuptake inhibitors (SSNRIs). Gabapentinoids are next to use.

Topical lidocaine should be considered alone or in combination with one the first-line therapies for localized peripheral neuropathic pain.

Opioid analgesics or tramadol could be used alone or in combination with one of the first-line therapies.

In painful diabetic peripheral neuropathy, gabapentinoids are recommended.

5. Medications used for pain and their pharmacologic properties in CKD patients

5.1. Acetaminophen

Acetaminophen, chemical name N-acetyl-p-aminophenol, is used as a first-line medication for mild and moderate pain. It is very well absorbed from the gastrointestinal tract, mainly in the small intestine, via passive transport, and its serum concentration peaks around 2 hours.

Any factors suppressing gastric emptying will slow paracetamol absorption, because negligible amount is absorbed in the stomach. It readily crosses the blood-brain barrier, and most antipyretic and analgesic actions are executed in the central nervous system.

Mechanism of action on receptors is not entirely made clear, but it has proposed actions on serotonergic pathways, potentiation of cannabinoid receptors, and inhibition of cyclooxygenase–3 and central prostaglandin production. Recent studies have questioned its biological activity regarding cyclooxygenase inhibition in peripheral tissues, and at least two recent studies experimentally proved that paracetamol possessed peripheral cyclooxygenase-2 inhibition [18–20].

Acetaminophen has been regarded as pain medication with very favorable side effect profile, when used within therapeutic range doses. But recently, some authors started to question its safety, especially possible association with kidney damage. In this study [21], CKD patients who were regularly taking acetaminophen were more likely to progress to ESRD, especially with increasing exposure. In another population-based, case-control study in Sweden, 926 patients were newly diagnosed with renal failure and acetaminophen was regularly consumed by 25% of them and only 12% of controls, and authors have concluded that the regular use of paracetamol increased the risk of CKD by 2.5 times from any cause [22]. Roberts et al. conducted systematic review of observational studies looking at acetaminophen's side effects, and they found increased relative rate of mortality from 0.95 to 1.63 and for cardiovascular adverse events risk ratio of all events increased from 1.19 to 1.68 and also that gastrointestinal adverse events or bleeds were found to increase from 1.11 to 1.49; moreover, kidney damage odds ratio increased more than 30% [23]. Another notable paper published on acetaminophen's cardiovascular side effect could only demonstrate small association with major cardiovascular events and short-term use of acetaminophen (odds ratio 1.21, 95% confidence interval 1.04–1.42) [24].

Acetaminophen's well-known hepatotoxicity occurs when the liver's glucuronide and sulfate stores are used up, forcing it to enter minor pathway, which is oxidation by CYP 450 enzymes and formation of N-acetyl-*p*-benzoquinone imine (NAPQI). This metabolite is harmless in the presence of glutathione but causes hepatotoxicity in patients with limited glutathione reserves.

The exact mechanisms for acetaminophen's renal toxicity have not been identified, whereas experimental research proposed that kidneys must be saturated and push acetaminophen via CYP 450 pathway for tubular damage to occur. Diminished glutathione reserve also exacerbated kidney toxicity [25]. Another possible mechanism is the formation of arylating intermediates by p-aminophenol, which is formed by deacetylation of acetaminophen [26]. Clinical manifestation of kidney injury appears as acute tubular necrosis, with corresponding urinary changes, such as granular casts, maybe with hematuria or pyuria, urine sodium increase, and azotemia as well [27]. Toxicity is exacerbated by factors such as fall in glutathione levels (any cachectic state, alcoholism) or induction of CYP 450 enzymes.

In normal conditions, plasma half-life of acetaminophen is 1.5–2.5 hours, large portion of which is metabolized and excreted in urine as sulfate and glucuronide conjugates, and minor pathway comprising less than 5% produces mercapturic and cysteine conjugates. Approximately 4% is excreted as unchanged drug. All of these processes will vary with age and dose administered. Urine flow rate is the main factor determining the clearance of acetaminophen by kidneys, but glucuronide and sulfate conjugates are not dependent of urine flow, most of the time surpassing glomerular filtration rate [28]. In CKD patients, it has been proved that glucuronide and sulfate metabolites are significantly accumulated, for example, in moderate stage of CKD, they have half-life around 21.8–30.5 hours as opposed to 3 hours in a normal person [29]. In ESRD patients undergoing dialysis, acetaminophen is removed by hemodialysis, but not by peritoneal dialysis.

Nonetheless, acetaminophen is still a preferred drug for mild to moderate pain, and no dose reductions are mandatory.

5.2. NSAIDs

NSAIDs as a group are highly unfavorable for any patient with kidney damage; nevertheless, many epidemiologic researchers have identified them as popular analgesics among CKD patients.

NSAIDs can be classified according to their chemical structure. They are divided into propionic acid derivatives (ibuprofen, ketoprofen, fenoprofen, naproxen), fenamates (diclofenac, ketorolac, tolmetin), enolic acid derivatives (meloxicam, piroxicam, nabumetone), and acetic acid derivatives (indomethacin, etodolac, sulindac). All these group medications inhibit the formation of prostaglandins in the peripheral tissues and, centrally, from arachidonic acid [30], hence exhibiting to different degrees analgesic, antipyretic, and anti-inflammatory effects. The action is achieved by blocking the cyclooxygenase (COX), which has two isoforms. COX-1 produces the group of prostaglandins which are necessary to maintain various physiological processes such as kidney function, maintenance of the gastrointestinal mucosa, and platelet aggregation. Yet, COX-2 is an inducible enzyme, production of which is prompted by inflammatory mediators (lipopolysaccharides, cytokines, and growth factors) by upregulating the expression of the enzyme up to 20-fold following the insult. Despite the fact that COX-2 is regarded as an inducible enzyme of inflammation process, the recent findings show that it plays an important role in normal physiology as well. It was found as an integral part of developing kidneys and brain, being a necessary enzyme for maturation and function. COX-2 maintains water electrolyte balance, contributes to arterial pressure regulation, and is mainly expressed in the thick ascending loop of Henle, macula densa of the nephron. The same enzyme is thought to play an important role in various tumor developments; especially it is overexpressed in intestinal adenomas, supporting many epidemiologic studies on the role of NSAIDs for colorectal cancer risk reduction.

Some authors believe that classification of NSAIDs should be according to their COX-2-to-COX-1 ratio, to better reflect their side effect profile [31], but along with inconsistent laboratory data, epidemiologic studies also show discrepancies in side effect profile of many NSAIDs. Instead, tabulating them according to half-life is of much clinical importance, which lets us to schedule medicine around the clock and avoid long-acting representatives in certain patients, including CKD patients. If the use of NSAIDs is required in CKD patients, preference should be given to those with short to medium half-life, such as ibuprofen, diclofenac, ketoprofen, and indomethacin, which have half-life less than 6 hours. Long-acting NSAIDs as naproxen, phenylbutazone, piroxicam, sulindac, diflunisal, and meloxicam (with half-life more than 10 hours) should be avoided.

Most of the NSAIDs have good bioavailability from the gastrointestinal tract, and their hepatic clearance is low. They also have almost equivalent efficacy, and most studies have demonstrated even comparable efficacy between nonspecific NSAIDs (nsNSAIDs) and coxibs [32]. Detailed pharmacokinetics of each NSAID is beyond the scope of this chapter; instead we will review their comparable side effect profile and application in CKD patients.

All NSAIDs possess to some extent of gastrointestinal, renal, and cardiovascular toxicities and fluid retention or aggravation of hypertension. Gastrointestinal toxicity is exacerbated by various additional risk factors such as preexisting *Helicobacter pylori* infection, advanced age, and the concomitant use of corticosteroids or aspirin. Coxibs are the least harmful to the gastrointestinal tract as compared to other nonselective NSAIDs, which increase the risk by 2–4 times [33]. The most hepatotoxic representatives are nimesulide, sulindac, and diclofenac [34].

The recent meta-analysis found that cardiovascular complications were significantly increased by both coxibs (rate ratio (RR) 1.37) and diclofenac (RR 1.41); the same analysis found ibuprofen increased coronary events significantly (RR 2.22), but naproxen was not found to contribute to major vascular events (RR 0.93). Heart failure risk was approximately increase by twofold by all representatives [33].

All NSAIDs, including coxibs, adversely affect kidney physiology, which is expected considering the important role that prostaglandins play in regulation of renal perfusion and filtration. These effects manifest as hypertension, fluid retention, and in severe cases acute kidney failure [30]. Exacerbating factors are preexisting kidney dysfunction and dehydration. But it is not clear if the chronic use of NSAIDs leads to CKD or worsens its course. Several recent epidemiologic studies tried to elucidate this matter. In one meta-analysis [35], authors have concluded that regular-dose NSAIDs were not found to exacerbate the advancement of CKD (OD = 0.96), but CKD accelerated with increased-dose NSAID use (OD = 1.26). And authors have concluded that it was acceptable to use NSAIDs in moderate to severe CKD, but doses must be tailored to minimal and effective at the same time.

In general, NSAIDs should be used in the short term and avoided in elderly, and precautions for gastric protection should be undertaken.

Despite well-known side effects and warnings, most of the CKD patients continue frequent consumption of NSAIDs, because these medications are easily available over the counter.

5.3. Opioids

The extent of opioid use among CKD patients is not well established. In recent review, it was reported to range around 18–36% [36].

As mentioned above, the use of opioids is highly undesirable in CKD patients, but in practice physicians are obliged to, due to the severity and poor pain control with non-opioid medications.

Morphine as a prototype opioid should be avoided as much as possible; it produces active metabolites which depend on kidney functions for clearance. The liver converts morphine to morphine-3-glucoronide approximately 55%, morphine-6-glucoronide 10%, and normorphine 4%.

In CKD patients accumulation of metabolites produces delayed suppression of respiratory drive; at the same time, other bothersome side effects such as pruritus can be challenging to manage. Morphine removed with hemodialysis up to 47%, but its metabolite, morphine-6-glucoronide, is fat-soluble and retained even after dialysis. It might be the cause of rebound phenomenon observed after dialysis.

Starting dose of morphine depends on glomerular filtration rate and should be around quarter to half of normal doses if it is 10–50 mL/min range and must be avoided at all if GFR is less than 10 mL/min.

Codeine is extensively metabolized to codeine-6-glucuronide (70%), to morphine by CYP2D6 enzymes (15%), and only 10–15% to norcodeine. About 5–15% of codeine is excreted by kidneys unchanged. Furthermore, morphine itself undergoes transformation to active metabolites as described above. All this makes codeine unsuitable for CKD patients; thus, no dosing regimen can be recommended at all.

Tramadol is known for its other, non-opioid properties, namely, inhibition of serotonin reuptake, which increases serotonin concentration in the synaptic cleft and low abuse potential. Tramadol produces active metabolites by O-demethylation (M1), which is more potent than tramadol itself and less active N,O-didesmethyltramadol (M5). These metabolites then undergo glucuronidation and are excreted by kidneys, 60% of initial dose as metabolites, and 30% unchanged. In CKD patients tramadol and its metabolites accumulate significantly, increasing the risk for respiratory depression and seizures, as well as serotonin syndrome. Recommended dose for tramadol in CKD patients with CrCl less than 30 mL/min is maximum of 100 mg twice daily and only 50 mg twice daily for stage 5 patients who are usually on dialysis [15].

Hydromorphone is considered relatively a better opioid option in CKD patients, despite the fact that it also produces active metabolite, hydromorphone-3-glucuronide, with seizure-inducing properties. This metabolite is removed via hemodialysis up to 40% [37]. Its analgesic properties are better than morphine, and some authors reported improvement of side effect profile, especially cognitive abilities after switching from morphine to hydromorphone [38]. Nevertheless, doses in CKD patients should be reduced, and dialysis patients should keep in mind that dialysis does not remove metabolites fully.

Oxycodone has same analgesic potency as morphine but better bioavailability and higher abuse potential. It is converted to inactive noroxycodone (45% of total dose) and active oxymorphone (19%). The latter is more potent than morphine with less pronounced side effects. Around 72%

is excreted via kidneys, of which 8% as oxycodone and the remaining as metabolites. In CKD patients, dose reduction is necessary, if GFR is less than 60 mL/min, the serum concentration of oxycodone reaches 50%; thus, starting dose should be 30% and titrated with lengthening the dosing interval. In stage 5 CKD patients, it is best to be avoided, although it is removed by dialysis.

Methadone was traditionally used in the treatment of opioid addiction but now increasingly prescribed for outpatient chronic pain patients. It has good bioavailability (mean value 75%), although pharmacokinetics greatly varies among individuals due to differences in CYP450 enzyme activity (which depends on genetics or patient's other medications). Eventually it undergoes N-demethylation in the liver by CYP3A4 to inactive metabolite. It has long life, elimination half-life reaching approximately 22 hours. Limited number of studies showed that no significant accumulation in CKD patients occurs, making it a suitable medication for renally impaired population. Therefore no dose adjustments are mandatory, except in cases when the patient is taking other CYP450-altering medications.

Buprenorphine is also extensively metabolized by the liver producing weak analgesic, norbuprenorphine. Thirty percent of both parent drug and metabolite is cleared by kidneys. In CKD patients, it can be used in regular doses in stages 1–4 but in stage 5 used with caution and monitoring. It is dialyzed by both hemo- and peritoneal dialysis.

Fentanyl is considered a safe opioid in CKD patients, and recommended route is transdermal patch (except in ESRD when it is avoided), but dose reduction should be up to 50% in severe to moderate CKD. It is mainly metabolized by oxidation in the liver, producing inactive metabolite, norfentanyl; 75% is excreted within 3 days. It is not dialyzed by either hemo- or peritoneal dialysis.

Alfentanil is similar to fentanyl, can be also used as a transdermal patch, and does not produce active metabolites. It is short and fast acting and also cannot be removed with dialysis. No dose reduction is required in CKD patients in any level.

When prescribing any opioid, all clinicians must follow safety precautions, explaining to patient treatment goals, using lowest dose to reach pain relief, following the patient regularly and frequent questioning of opioid need.

6. Non-pharmacological pain control

Non-pharmacological approach to pain management starts with working on psychological components of the pain. Devine et al. analyzed 191 studies and confirmed significance of psychological and educational care of surgical patients and its role in managing acute postoperative pain. It included providing patients with proper information about procedures and the expected level of pain, instructing them on proper coughing and breathing techniques, and providing emotional support [39].

Transition from acute to chronic pain conditions also involves several psychological factors such as depressive state, somatization, or significant distress [40].

Many kinds of questionnaires and tests were developed to be applied in chronic pain, discussion of which is beyond the scope of this chapter. Generally, psychological management of chronic pain patients should be carried out with the help of certified psychologist or psychiatrist.

http://dx.doi.org/10.5772/intechopen.81695

Considering the burden of musculoskeletal pain in CKD patients, therapies to reduce muscle tension and myofascial release should be applied, such as bed rest, bracing, traction, manipulation and mobilization, exercise, and heat/cold applications. Acupuncture was proven to be effective in lower back pain and knee pain; therefore, along with mindfulness, meditation and relaxation techniques prove to be safe and applicable to CKD patients too [41].

7. Conclusion

A considerable number of CKD patients experience acute pain at some point of their life, and even bigger portion of this population suffer from chronic pain. It is apparent from epidemiologic studies that pain can be experienced by more than 50% of CKD patients and greatly affects their quality of life. Moreover, poor pain control may lead to exacerbation of other psychological symptoms and contribute to further patient deterioration. If it is relatively clear how to manage acute pain in hospitalized patients, chronic pain remains mostly understudied and not fully understood. WHO stepwise approach to treating cancer pain may be tailored to CKD patients considering disturbances of pharmacodynamics of most medications in renal impairment. When there is a need to prescribe opioids, all precautions for side effects and addiction prevention must be taken. Pain practitioners should actively advocate non-pharmacological pain management techniques in appropriate patients.

Conflict of interest

Nothing to declare.

Author details

Shakhsanam Mirishova* and Yasser Mahmoud Hammad Ali Hammad

*Address all correspondence to: smirishova@hamad.qa

Hamad Medical Corporation, Doha, Qatar

References

[1] Murtagh FE, Addington-Hall JM, Edmonds PM, Donohoe P, Carey I, Jenkins K, et al. Symptoms in advanced renal disease: A cross-sectional survey of symptom prevalence in stage 5 chronic kidney disease managed without dialysis. Journal of Palliative Medicine. 2007;**10**(6):1266-1276

[2] Davison SN, Koncicki H, Brennan F. Pain in chronic kidney disease: A scoping review. Seminars in Dialysis. 2014;**27**(2):188-204

[3] Brown SA, Tyrer FC, Clarke AL, Lloyd-Davies LH, Stein AG, Tarrant C, et al. Symptom burden in patients with chronic kidney disease not requiring renal replacement therapy. Clinical Kidney Journal. 2017;**10**(6):788-796

[4] Perlman RL, Finkelstein FO, Liu L, Roys E, Kiser M, Eisele G, et al. Quality of life in chronic kidney disease (CKD): A cross-sectional analysis in the Renal Research Institute-CKD study. American Journal of Kidney Diseases. 2005;**45**(4):658-666

[5] Davison SN. Pain in hemodialysis patients: Prevalence, cause, severity, and management. American Journal of Kidney Diseases. 2003;**42**(6):1239-1247

[6] Weisbord SD, Fried LF, Arnold RM, Fine MJ, Levenson DJ, Peterson RA, et al. Prevalence, severity, and importance of physical and emotional symptoms in chronic hemodialysis patients. Journal of the American Society of Nephrology. 2005;**16**(8):2487-2494

[7] Davison SN, Jhangri GS. Impact of pain and symptom burden on the health-related quality of life of hemodialysis patients. Journal of Pain and Symptom Management. 2010;**39**(3):477-485

[8] National Kidney Foundation. K/DOQI clinical practice guidelines for chronic kidney disease: Evaluation, classification, and stratification. American Journal of Kidney Diseases. 2002;**39**(2 Suppl 1):S1-S266

[9] Tawfic QA, Bellingham G. Postoperative pain management in patients with chronic kidney disease. Journal of Anaesthesiology Clinical Pharmacology. 2015;**31**(1):6-13. DOI: 10.4103/0970-9185.150518

[10] Dauri M, Faria S, Gatti A, Celidonio L, Carpenedo R, Sabato AF. Gabapentin and pregabalin for the acute post-operative pain management. A systematic-narrative review of the recent clinical evidences. Current Drug Targets. 2009;**10**:716-733

[11] Andersohn F, Suissa S, Garbe E. Use of first- and second-generation cyclooxygenase-2-selective nonsteroidal anti-inflammatory drugs and risk of acute myocardial infarction. Circulation. 2006;**113**(16):1950-1957

[12] Murtagh FE, Chai MO, Donohoe P, Edmonds PM, Higginson IJ. The use of opioid analgesia in end-stage renal disease patients managed without dialysis: Recommendations for practice. Journal of Pain & Palliative Care Pharmacotherapy. 2007;**21**:5-16

[13] Bonica JJ. The Management of Pain. Philadelphia: Lea & Febiger; 1953

[14] Treede RD, Rief W, Barke A, Aziz Q, Bennett MI, Benoliel R, et al. A classification of chronic pain for ICD-11. Pain. 2015;**156**(6):1003-1007

[15] Pham PC, Khaing K, Sievers TM, Pham PM, Miller JM, Pham SV, et al. 2017 update on pain management in patients with chronic kidney disease. Clinical Kidney Journal. 2017;**10**(5):688-697

[16] World Health Organization. Cancer Pain Relief: With a Guide to Opioid Availability. 2nd ed. Geneva: World Health Organization; 1996. pp. 3-36

[17] Goldberg RJ, Katz J. A meta-analysis of the analgesic effects of omega-3 polyunsaturated fatty acid supplementation for inflammatory joint pain. Pain. 2007;**129**:210-223

[18] Brune K, Renner B, Tiegs G. Acetaminophen/paracetamol: A history of errors, failures and false decisions. European Journal of Pain. 2015;**19**(7):953-965

[19] Hinz B, Cheremina O, Brune K. Acetaminophen (paracetamol) is a selective cyclooxygenase-2 inhibitor in man. The FASEB Journal. 2008;**22**(2):383-390

[20] Lee YS, Kim H, Brahim JS, Rowan J, Lee G, Dionne RA. Acetaminophen selectively suppresses peripheral prostaglandin E2 release and increases COX-2 gene expression in a clinical model of acute inflammation. Pain. 2007;**129**(3):279-286

[21] Kuo HW, Tsai SS, Tiao MM, Liu YC, Lee IM, Yang CY. Analgesic use and the risk for progression of chronic kidney disease. Pharmacoepidemiology and Drug Safety. 2010;**19**(7):745-751

[22] Fored CM, Ejerblad E, Lindblad P, Fryzek JP, Dickman PW, Signorello LB, et al. Acetaminophen, aspirin, and chronic renal failure. The New England Journal of Medicine. 2001;**345**(25):1801-1808

[23] Roberts E, Delgado Nunes V, Buckner S, Latchem S, Constanti M, Miller P, et al. Paracetamol: Not as safe as we thought? A systematic literature review of observational studies. Annals of the Rheumatic Diseases. 2016;**75**:552-559

[24] Gonzalez-Valcarcel J, Sissani L, Labreuche J, Bousser MG, Chamorro A, Fisher M, et al. Paracetamol, ibuprofen, and recurrent major cardiovascular and major bleeding events in 19120 patients with recent ischemic stroke. Stroke. 2016;**47**(4):1045-1052

[25] Mitchell JR, McMurtry RJ, Statham CN, Nelson SD. Molecular basis for several drug-induced nephropathies. The American Journal of Medicine. 1977;**62**(4):518-526

[26] Newton JF, Pasino DA, Hook JB. Acetaminophen nephrotoxicity in the rat: Quantitation of renal metabolic activation in vivo. Toxicology and Applied Pharmacology. 1985; **78**(1):39-46

[27] Blakely P, McDonald BR. Acute renal failure due to acetaminophen ingestion: A case report and review of the literature. Journal of the American Society of Nephrology. 1995; **6**(1):48-53

[28] Prescott LF. Kinetics and metabolism of paracetamol and phenacetin. British Journal of Clinical Pharmacology. 1980;**10**(Suppl 2):291S-298S

[29] Prescott LF, Speirs GC, Critchley JA, Temple RM, Winney RJ. Paracetamol disposition and metabolite kinetics in patients with chronic renal failure. European Journal of Clinical Pharmacology. 1989;**36**(3):291-297

[30] Hemmings HC, Egan TD. Pharmacology and Physiology for Anesthesia: Foundations and Clinical Application. Philadelphia, PA: Elsevier, Inc; 2013

[31] Frolich JC. A classification of NSAIDs according to the relative inhibition of cyclooxygenase isoenzymes. Trends in Pharmacological Sciences. 1997;**18**(1):30-34

[32] Singh G, Fort JG, Goldstein JL, Levy RA, Hanrahan PS, Bello AE, et al. Celecoxib versus naproxen and diclofenac in osteoarthritis patients: SUCCESS-I study. The American Journal of Medicine. 2006;**119**(3):255-266

[33] Bhala N, Emberson J, Merhi A, Abramson S, Arber N, Baron JA, et al. Vascular and upper gastrointestinal effects of non-steroidal anti-inflammatory drugs: Meta-analyses of individual participant data from randomised trials. Lancet. 2013;**382**(9894):769-779

[34] Aithal GP, Day CP. Nonsteroidal anti-inflammatory drug-induced hepatotoxicity. Clinics in Liver Disease. 2007;**11**(3):563-575. vi-vii

[35] Nderitu P, Doos L, Jones PW, Davies SJ, Kadam UT. Non-steroidal anti-inflammatory drugs and chronic kidney disease progression: A systematic review. Family Practice. 2013;**30**(3):247-255

[36] Nagar VR, Birthi P, Salles S, Sloan PA. Opioid use in chronic pain patients with chronic kidney disease: A systematic review. Pain Medicine. 2017;**18**(8):1416-1449

[37] Durnin C, Hind ID, Wickens MM, Yates DB, Molz KH. Pharmacokinetics of oral immediate-release hydromorphone (Dilaudid IR) in subjects with renal impairment. Proceedings of the Western Pharmacology Society. 2001;**44**:81-82

[38] Lee MA, Leng ME, Tiernan EJ. Retrospective study of the use of hydromorphone in palliative care patients with normal and abnormal urea and creatinine. Palliative Medicine. 2001;**15**(1):26-34

[39] Devine EC. Effects of psychoeducational care for adult surgical patients: A meta-analysis of 191 studies. Patient Education and Counseling. 1992;**19**(2):129-142

[40] Pincus T, Burton AK, Vogel S, Field AP. A systematic review of psychological factors as predictors of chronicity/disability in prospective cohorts of low back pain. Spine. 2002;**27**(5):E109-E120

[41] Tick H, Nielsen A, Pelletier KR, Bonakdar R, Simmons S, Glick R, et al. Evidence-based nonpharmacologic strategies for comprehensive pain care: The consortium pain task force white paper. Explorer. 2018;**14**(3):177-211

Chapter 7

Management of Acute Pain in Obese Patients with Sleep Apnea

Sayed Rahman, Ahmed Zaghw, Osama Elazzouny,
Dhari Almenshid, Mustafa Rezk,
Mohammed Azizuddin Imran and Malek Alali

Additional information is available at the end of the chapter

http://dx.doi.org/10.5772/intechopen.80350

Abstract

Perioperative pain management for obese patients is daily challenges for anesthesiologists especially if complex comorbidities such as Obstructive Sleep Apnea and cardiovascular disease coexist. Limitations to effective pain management in this group are multifactorial, that includes technical difficulty with regional techniques, limited expertise, unavailability of standardized guidelines and lack of familiarity with recent multimodal analgesic regimens. Opioid-related complications such as narcotic-induced ventilatory depression in these group of patients poses another critical concern for both trainees and the experienced anesthesiologists. This chapter is intended for residents, fellows, as well as senior perioperative physicians, and will explore various regional and pharmacological options for acute pain management in this special population based on recent advances and available evidence.

Keywords: acute pain, obstructive sleep apnea (OSA), OSA pathology, opioid interaction with OSA, multimodal pain management

1. Introduction

Obesity is one of the growing worldwide epidemics that has doubled since 1980. In 2016, about 39% of women and men across the world were overweight, and 11% of men and 15% of women were obese [1]. Obesity is a chronic systemic disease characterized by abnormal and excessive fat deposition with a significant impact on individual's quality of life and life expectancy in addition to its burden on public health resources. Overweight and obesity are defined as BMI ≥ 25 kg/m^2 and ≥ 30 kg/m^2, respectively. Beyond that BMI-centric definition, complications-centric approach is more comprehensive and clinically relevant to assess the adiposity-based chronic disease (ABCD). Airway obstruction is a common comorbidity in the obese population, with an estimated prevalence of 40% in moderate obesity, and up to 90% in patients with severe obesity. The grade of airway obstruction proportionally correlates with the severity of obesity. It has been shown that each 1-SD increase in BMI increases the risk of OSA four folds [2], moreover a 10% change in body weight increases the severity of OSA by 30%, as measured by apnea–hypopnea index [3]. OSA on top of obesity is associated with worse perioperative outcomes in terms of difficult intubation, postoperative respiratory, atrial fibrillation and other perioperative cardiac events [4]. Given the increasing prevalence of obesity, anesthesiologists are very likely to find themselves caring for obese patients with sleep apnea. This necessitates anesthesiologists and pain physicians to acquire a clear understanding of OSA pathology, familiarity with multimodal pain modalities, experience with regional anesthesia and structured pain management protocols. This chapter is an OSA-centered review of the commonly used pain medications and the most clinically relevant topics in OSA pathology and pain management. It is intended to be a quick review for residents, fellows in training and pain physicians and is equipped with the latest evidence-based management options.

2. Obstructive sleep apnea

Obstructive Sleep Apnea (OSA) is one of four types of breathing problems that occur during sleep. These include sleep apnea due to a central cause, hypoventilation, and hypoxemia during sleep. OSA presents as daytime sleepiness, loud snoring, witnessed apneic episodes, or frequent awakenings due to airway obstruction. In OSA, at least one of the obstructive respiratory events such as apneas, hypopneas or increased respiratory effort related arousals occur per hour of sleep. The alternating episodes of snoring and silence lasting 20–30 seconds are usually associated with a reduction in blood oxygen saturation and interruption of sleep pattern [5]. Risk factors include obesity, male gender and postmenopausal state [6]. It is prevalent in 4% of men and 2% of women, with predominance in 40–60 years of age. It is believed that the number of patients suffering from OSA is underestimated, given the lack of an accurate screening tool [6]. The National Sleep Foundation (NSF) found 26% of American healthy adults at a high risk of OSA based on Berlin questionnaire assessment [6].

OSA could be mild, moderate or severe, depending upon the respiratory disturbance index (RDI). RDI between 5 and 15 is mild, between 16 and 30 is moderate and more than 30 per hour is severe [5, 7]. The severity of OSA requires an objective testing with sleep study using polysomnography or portable monitors at home or drug induced sleep endoscopy (DISE), as it impacts treatment decisions.

3. OSA pathophysiology and its interaction with opioid pharmacology

OSA is a systemic disease with multiorgan involvement that is not limited to obstruction of the upper airways. It is associated with significant negative functional and cognitive outcomes apart from a higher morbidity and mortality. OSA is associated with cardiovascular morbidities including pulmonary and systemic hypertension, heart disease, ischemic stroke, diabetes and metabolic syndrome [8–12]. During sleep, OSA patients have depressed ventilation, which worsens with any perioperative opioids. It is known that arousal is a protective mechanism.

OSA is the result of interaction between normal sleep physiology and abnormal upper airway anatomy. The narrowing of upper airways can be due to either soft tissues or bony structures. Soft tissues factors include an enlarged tongue, increased soft tissue volume, fat deposition in upper airways or enlarged tonsils in pediatric patients. The latter can be heritable and seen in the absence of obesity [13]. Bony structures can also affect patency of the airway. Increased mandibular length was associated with less risk for OSA development in male individuals [14]. Patients with OSA tend to have an impaired arousal in response to airway obstruction [15].

REM stage of sleep causes a generalized loss of muscle tone including muscles responsible for patency of the upper airway; genioglossus, palatal muscles and hyoid muscles [6–8]. Under physiological conditions, sleep causes narrowed airway caliber, increased airway resistance and increased upper airway compliance [16, 17]. This could increase the work of breathing causing hypoventilation and increased arterial partial pressure of carbon dioxide ($PaCO_2$). During wakefulness, the decreased airflow through a narrowed airway is compensated by increasing respiratory muscle effort thus creating greater negative intrathoracic pressure, a reflex known as mechanical load compensation [18]. This mechanism is normally lost during sleep and is more exaggerated in OSA patients.

Such physiologic changes during sleep may be well tolerated in individuals with an acceptable airway anatomy. But with an already narrowed upper airway, sleep-induced hypotonia can potentially cause complete obstruction of the airway. The interaction between these physiologic and pathologic factors leads to recurrent airway collapse resulting in reduced (hypopnea) or complete cessation of airflow (apnea) despite patient's breathing efforts. This eventually leads to intermittent blood gas disturbances (hypoxia and hypercapnia) and interrupted sleep. The typical feature of OSA is a cyclic breathing pattern that develops, with alternating cycles of obstructive breathing events (sleep) and arousal (wakefulness).

Breathing during sleep is dependent on the chemoreceptor and mechanoreceptor inputs to the brain. Hypoxia and hypercapnia stimulate the central chemoreceptors and peripheral carotid and aortic bodies chemoreceptors which in turn stimulate ventilation and cause cortical arousal. Increased respiratory muscle effort per se can cause cortical arousal [19]. Once arousal occurs, inspiratory upper motor neurons are stimulated resulting in a rapid recovery of dilator muscle activity, return of muscular tone in the genioglossus and pharyngeal muscles with resulting relief of airway obstruction [20, 21].This subsequently leads to restoration of blood oxygen levels and clearance of the accumulated carbon dioxide. When the patient falls asleep, the cycle of obstruction and hypoxia recurs and so on. Arousal is the predominant protective mechanism in OSA, after which oxygen and carbon dioxide levels return to normal. All of the opioids cause varying degrees of sedation and sleep-disordered breathing, that could be central sleep apnea and peripheral OSA [22, 23]. As patients with OSA are at a higher risk of oxygen desaturation, opioids sparing analgesic techniques are preferred [24].

4. Causes of acute pain in patients with OSA

Patients with OSA may experience acute pain in a nonsurgical or a surgical setting. Listed below in **Table 1** are some of the common causes:

Nonsurgical causes	1.	**Headache**: mostly morning headache, very common, 50% of OSA patients [25], unknown cause.
	2.	**Coronary artery disease (CAD)**: OSA is associated with higher thrombotic risk [26].
	3.	**Tonsillitis**: pain and difficulty in swallowing [27].
Common surgical causes	1.	**Tonsillectomy**: "Post-tonsillectomy pain" due to disruption of mucosa and glossopharyngeal nerve irritation the pharyngeal muscles spasms [28].
	2.	**Uvulopalatoplasty**: [29].
	3.	**Bariatric surgery**: laparoscopic bariatric surgeries which are less painful than open surgeries [30].

Table 1. Some common causes of acute pain in patients with OSA.

5. Drug treatment options

The choice of one analgesic over the others is dependent on its safety profile and the interaction with OSA and its complications. Interestingly, the systemic effects of OSA like chronic hypoxemia and systemic inflammation can increase analgesic sensitivity to opioids [31]. Chronic intermittent hypoxemia activates hypoxemia inducible factor-1 alpha which in turn increases expression of mu opioid receptor and delta opioid receptor expression, augmenting opioid sensitivity [32].

5.1. Opioid medications

5.1.1. Opioid effects on ventilation

Opioids depresses the respiratory drive by inhibition of respiratory centers in the brain stem, thus decreasing the respiratory rate and the tidal volume [33]. Opioids could also obstruct the upper airway through loss of muscle tone due to sedation or through direct inhibition of central neurons responsible for maintaining upper airway muscle tone [34]. Moreover, it alters the upper airway reflexes and responses to ventilatory depression [35].

The respiratory depression results in hypoventilation with subsequent increase in $PaCO_2$ [33]. These effects are dose-dependent and could be life-threatening with higher doses of opioids or multiple boluses that are commonly used in perioperative period or after major trauma. Those additive risks in OSA patients with already depressed ventilation and airway obstruction could increase the risk of respiratory events and mortality after recovery from anesthesia. Therefore, it is prudent to start with the lowest dose recommended and carefully titrate to effect.

5.1.2. Opioid-induced sleep disturbances

Patients without OSA who are on chronic opioid therapy have been reported to have sleep disturbances, impaired self-reported sleep and poor sleep quality [36]. These effects might exacerbate already disturbed sleep in OSA patients.

5.1.3. Opioid effects on the cardiovascular system

Opioids have unfavorable hemodynamic effects in OSA patients such as hypotension, orthostatic hypotension, and syncope of various degrees. The negative hemodynamic effects are due to central vasomotor depression, direct myocardial depression, and arteriovenous dilatation in higher doses [37]. In general, cautious use of opioids should be considered in patients with severe OSA associated with hypertension, arrhythmias and heart failure. Fentanyl has a relatively favorable cardiovascular profile compared to other opioids. For anesthetic management, it has modest effects on blood pressure and myocardial contractility. It is well tolerated as an analgesic regarding cardiovascular adverse effects compared with other opioids. Morphine has the greatest potential for histamine release, compared to other opioids, resulting in hypotension. Hydromorphone can cause a greater drop-in blood pressure compared to equipotent doses of morphine. Tramadol has a lower risk of cardiovascular adverse events, but it can lead to serotonin syndrome and cardiac arrhythmias. Meperidine administration leads to significant decrease in blood pressure and cardiac output due to direct myocardial depressant effects and peripheral vasodilatation. It can predispose patients to serotonin crisis [38]. Methadone is recently becoming popular in chronic pain management. However, it has been associated with QTc prolongation with a risk of torsade de pointes [35, 39].

5.2. Nonsteroidal anti-inflammatory drugs (NSAIDs)

These are foundational analgesics and highly effective as they have lower numbers needed to treat (NNT) comparable with other medications. Ketorolac and Ibuprofen are the commonly used NSAIDs in a perioperative setting. The American Society of Anesthesiologists (ASA) taskforce recommends the use of perioperative NSAIDs to decrease narcotic consumption [40]. A reduction in narcotic consumption in the postsurgical period was achieved by regular administration of Ketorolac in morbidly obese patients [41, 42]. Likewise, intravenous intraoperative Ketorolac infusion has been shown to reduce pain scores in the same population [42]. NSAIDs should be used with caution in patients with hypertension, arrhythmias, heart failure and chronic kidney disease. They can increase the risk of serious cardiovascular events, myocardial ischemia, and stroke and the risk is proportional to the duration of their use. Selective COX 2 inhibitors carry a higher risk than nonselective COX inhibitors. If NSAIDs use is necessary for high-risk patients, it is advisable to use the lowest dose possible for the shortest duration. NSAIDs could precipitate acute kidney injury in patients with compensated heart failure or diabetic nephropathy and also further worsen underlying chronic kidney disease (CKD) [43, 44]. The hyperkalemia is mild, but could be critical in patients with elevated K^+ serum levels due to CKD or with concomitant use of ACE inhibitors. The inhibition of platelet aggregation through decreased production of thromboxane A_2 could potentially increase bleeding in patients already on anticoagulants.

5.3. Acetaminophen

Acetaminophen is a commonly used foundational analgesic with perioperative opioid sparing properties. It offers the distinct advantage of being relatively safe and devoid of sedative properties. Addition of acetaminophen to an intravenous opioid PCA regimen was associated with a 20% opioid sparing effect in a meta-analysis of mixed surgical population [45]. Similar opioid dose reduction expected in patients with OSA could therefore potentially reduce opioid-induced ventilator problems. Obese bariatric surgical patients receiving postoperative intravenous acetaminophen 1 gram every 6 hours required fewer morphine equivalents [46]. Acetaminophen lowers cumulative narcotic consumption, regardless of the route of administration [47, 48]. It has the most favorable effect on blood pressure and should be considered as the first line treatment option in patients with hypertension or cardiovascular disease.

5.4. Anticonvulsant agents

Anticonvulsant agents in clinical use for their analgesic benefits include Pregabalin and Gabapentin. The preoperative use of Pregabalin as premedication significantly lowered immediate postoperative requirement of pain medications among bariatric surgical patients. [49] Preoperative Gabapentin has also significantly lowered immediate postoperative pain scores in morbidly obese bariatric surgical patients [50]. However, the most common side effects of these drugs are dizziness and somnolence, which potentially add to the OSA induced somnolence. Postoperative respiratory depression with the use of Pregabalin has been reported in a patient with undiagnosed obstructive sleep apnea [51]. Concomitant opioid use could increase the risk of respiratory depression and caution should be considered. The Ottawa hospital algorithm for Pregabalin use recommends either avoiding or cautiously titrating low doses depending on the clinical setting and patient characteristics [51]. Pregabalin and Gabapentin could cause peripheral edema which is not related to cardiac, hepatic or kidney failure [52].

5.5. Alpha $_2$ agonists

Alpha $_2$ agonists such as Clonidine and Dexmedetomidine are used in perioperative setting for their analgesic properties. A meta-analysis conducted in a mixed general surgical population suggested that perioperative alpha $_2$ agonists reduce narcotic consumption in the postoperative period [53]. However, very limited data is available regarding their use in obese patients with OSA. Nonopioid anesthetic with Dexmedetomidine in obese patients with OSA resulted in low pain scores in Post Anesthesia Care Unit (PACU) and no perioperative events [54]. Among patients with morbid obesity, substitution of intraoperative opioids with an intraoperative Dexmedetomidine infusion resulted in reduced perioperative opioid requirements [55]. Also, perioperative Dexmedetomidine infusion were found to significantly reduce postoperative opioid consumption (24-hours) as compared to conventional perioperative analgesic regimens [56]. Alpha $_2$ agonists can cause sedation which could interfere with arousal in OSA patients. However, their opioid sparing benefits may offer greater benefit than the risks. Clonidine causes adverse effects like hypotension, bradycardia, sinus and AV nodal block [57]. Dexmedetomidine causes hypotension and bradycardia more often than hypertension

http://dx.doi.org/10.5772/intechopen.80350

and tachycardia. It may also reduce atrial fibrillation (AF) induction among adult patients with history of paroxysmal AF.

5.6. Ketamine

Ketamine, an *N*-methyl-d-aspartate (NMDA) antagonist has recently received increasing attention as a relatively safe adjuvant analgesic. In patients with morbid obesity, low-dose Ketamine added to intravenous Morphine PCA resulted in a significant reduction in opioid consumption. Importantly, subjects receiving ketamine in addition to morphine had fewer episodes of desaturation postoperatively [9]. A preinduction dose of ketamine of 0.5 mg kg^{-1} together with Clonidine significantly lowered pain scores and perioperative opioids consumed [58]. Intra-operative Ketamine at doses up to 1 mg kg^{-1} was shown to decrease opioid consumption in recovery but at the cost of significant drowsiness [59].

5.7. Tramadol

It is an analgesic of intermediate potency with possible advantages in OSA patients due to its multimodal mechanism and a relatively lower risk of respiratory depression [60].

6. Multimodal strategies for pain management in obese patients with OSA

Multimodal analgesia is the use of a combination of different analgesic medications and techniques with an aim to provide optimal pain control, thus allowing reduction in opioid requirements. They may have additive or synergistic effects by acting through diverse mechanisms either peripherally or centrally in the nervous system [61]. Multimodal analgesia with a combination of IV Paracetamol and IV Ketorolac in bariatric surgery was found to reduce the postoperative opioid consumption by about 70% [62]. A nonopioid analgesic regimen that employed a combination of nonopioid analgesics (Ketorolac, Clonidine, Ketamine, Lidocaine and Magnesium) in thirty morbidly obese patients undergoing bariatric surgery resulted in lesser PACU opioid consumption and less sedation [63]. The opioid-sparing multimodal techniques are summarized in **Table 2**.

Magnesium, intravenous local anesthetic infusions (lidocaine), and Clonidine are some additional drugs that have been used perioperatively in patients with morbid obesity to enhance analgesia [64, 65] but more scientific evidence is needed before adopting these agents into routine clinical use.

6.1. Regional analgesia techniques in patients with obstructive sleep apnea

Narcotic-based pain regimens for OSA patients have a risk of opioid-induced respiratory depression. Hypoxia, sleep disturbance, pain, and disturbed opioid responses in OSA contribute to that risk [66, 67]. Neuraxial techniques and peripheral nerve blocks are effective

Nonopioid analgesics include
Nonsteroidal anti-inflammatory drugs (NSAIDs),
Acetaminophen,
Analgesic adjuvants such as Ketamine, Dexmedetomidine, and Clonidine may also decrease postoperative opioid requirements.
Regional analgesia with local anesthetic (e.g., peripheral nerve blocks, epidural analgesia)

Table 2. Opioid-sparing techniques include a combination of the following.

interventions and superior alternatives in pain management toolkits. It offers a superior analgesic effect and minimizes the need for systemic analgesics [68, 69].

Perioperative management by regional analgesic techniques rather than systemic opioids has been recommended by the American Society of Anesthesiologists since 2014, with an aim to reduce the likelihood of OSA-related perioperative adverse outcomes. The beneficial effects of perioperative regional analgesic techniques on patient outcomes have been proved in general surgical population [70, 71]. Still, the evidence in OSA patients is inconclusive as it was driven mainly from case reports or small retrospective case–control studies [67, 72].

6.2. Neuraxial analgesia techniques

Neuraxial analgesia is a modality with high efficacy and can be used effectively as a sole analgesic approach. Its beneficial effects on respiratory functions such as superior spirometry in the immediate postoperative period and lower postoperative pulmonary complications have been consistently documented in many studies [73, 74]. The risks in morbidly obese patients include respiratory depression secondary to a rostral spread of neuraxial opioids that could lead to a postoperative respiratory arrest [75, 76]. Therefore, the ASA task force recommends that expected benefits should be weighed against the potential risks.

Technical difficulty with procedure failure has been proposed as another challenge in OSA patients, who are often obese. Yet, these concerns lack conclusive evidence, and most have been driven from opinion-based reports. Studies in obese pregnant have showed that the incidence of technical difficulty for epidural anesthesia is overrated. The success was correlated with optimal positioning prior to placement and good quality of palpable surface landmarks [77]. Preprocedural ultrasonography (US) of the spine could accurately identify the intervertebral space and predict the needle insertion depth in intrathecal space thus facilitating placement of an epidural catheter. Systematic review and meta-analysis have shown that spine US has a greater accuracy than manual palpation of surface anatomical landmarks [78]. This could lead to a decreased risk of technical failures and the number of needle punctures.

6.3. Peripheral nerve blocks (PNB)

PNB modality is another pillar of opioid-sparing analgesic techniques. It includes upper extremity, lower extremity, and planar blocks such as transversus abdominis plane (TAP) block, paravertebral block, and erector spinae plane block (ESP). Initially, studies showed that obesity (BMI > 25 kg/m^2) is independent risk factor for block failure. [45] However, other studies showed not much of a difference in success rate between obese and nonobese and proved that success mainly depends on experience of anesthesiologist and the use of ultrasound-guided techniques [46]. Upper extremity blocks include brachial plexus block that could be performed at different levels. It offers good analgesia for patients with OSA who have a respiratory compromise. Phrenic nerve block is a theoretical risk with inter-scalene block. There is insufficient evidence to recommend its use in this group of patients [79]. Ultrasound-guided transversus abdominis plane (TAP) block is performed in laparoscopic and open abdominal surgeries as it effectively blocks T10 to L1 segments. A successful bilateral TAP block is effective for abdominal midline incisions, especially in nonobese and in situations of failed or difficult epidurals [63]. Paravertebral block is another option for thoracoabdominal surgeries. It could be administered as a single shot or continuous technique, either intra or postoperatively. Multilevel paravertebral block has shown to be successful and opioid-sparing in obese females undergoing breast surgery [80]. The erector spinae plane block (ESP) is a recently evolved simple technique that could be performed under ultrasound guidance. It is gaining popularity for its effective pain relief for somatic and visceral pain. However, further clinical investigation is needed to clearly establish its efficacy in OSA patients. Perioperative analgesia for OSA patients could be carefully planned in the perioperative period. Many effective regional analgesia modalities are currently available for intraoperative and postoperative.

7. Combined strategies for analgesia

Preemptive analgesia could obtund nociceptive responses prior to surgical stimulus and possibly decrease postoperative pain. Moreover, it could possibly decrease the probability of conversion of acute pain to chronic pain [81]. Postoperative patient-controlled intravenous analgesia (PCA) or epidural analgesia (PCEA) have been shown to decrease narcotic consumption and provide a high degree of patient satisfaction [82]. Other techniques like long-acting local anesthetic infusions at the surgical wound site or even intraperitoneal infusion have shown promising results [83, 84].

Poor pain management of morbidly obese patients increases postoperative complications [85]. Therefore, the use of multimodal analgesia can solve this problem, consequently improving patient satisfaction and reduce postoperative morbidity.

Developing an optimal evidence-based pain management protocol tailored to obese patients with OSA is a challenging task. The majority of current recommendations are either based on studies with small sample size or lacking a scientifically rigorous study design. Given the paucity of literature in obese patients with sleep apnea, it is difficult to draw a definitive conclusion. Yet, the obvious benefits of multimodal analgesic regimen make it popular in regular clinical practice.

8. Nonpharmacological options to pain management

The nonpharmacological options are summarized in **Table 3:**

Peripheral therapies (physical skin stimulation)	
Transcutaneous electrical nerve stimulation (TENS)	Application of electricity to stimulate the skin can be used to manage different types of pain. The mechanism could possibly be explained by Gate control theory. There is a lack of strong evidence to suggest benefits of TENS in labor pain
Hot-cold treatment	Can be used in acute musculoskeletal injury [86].
Acupuncture and acupressure	It could reduce cancer pain intensity [87]
Exercise	To relieve pain by preventing spasms and contractures [13].
Positioning	Adequate position in the postoperative period by pillows and special beds. [13]
Restriction of movement/resting	Prolonged bed rest is not recommended—the bed rest for about two days may be beneficial after back surgeries by reducing edema.
Cognitive-behavioral therapies	
Distraction by music	Decreases pain sensitivity and increase pain tolerance
Reflexology	Special techniques employed to apply pressure at reflex points on feet corresponding to various body parts decreases pain perception by altering physiology [13].
Meditation, Yoga, Hypnosis, Herbal treatments, Aromatherapy, Relaxation—respiration techniques	

Table 3. Summarization of the nonpharmacological options.

9. Monitoring, oxygen and positive airway pressure therapy for obese patients with sleep apnea

9.1. Monitoring

Oxygen saturation and respiratory rate should be closely monitored in these group of patients receiving opioids or other potentially sedative medications [88]. For continuous assessment of the adequacy of ventilation in the postoperative setting, end-tidal CO_2 measurement has become the standard of care [89, 90]. End-tidal CO_2 detects hypoventilation earlier than any other physiological monitors. OSA patients at high risk should be continuously monitored with pulse oximetry until patient maintains oxygen saturation to their preoperative baseline levels [91, 92]. Studies have shown that pulse oximetry monitoring in postoperative patients is very useful in detecting hypoxemic episodes [40, 93].

9.2. Oxygen therapy

Obese patients with suspected or confirmed OSA should be transferred with supplemental oxygen from operation room to the post-anesthesia care unit (PACU) after receiving general anesthesia. In the PACU, patient head end elevation by at least 30 degrees is recommended. Though there is not enough literature that shows the effect of supplemental oxygen in postoperative settings, the recommendation is that supplemental oxygen should be continued in all postoperative OSA patients until they maintain preoperative (baseline) oxygen saturation on room air [91].

9.3. Positive airway pressure therapy

Use of CPAP in PACU is recommended for OSA patients who were using it preoperatively at home and also when patients get frequent attacks of airway obstruction in the recovery room [91, 94]. It should also be continued on the inpatient units. CPAP has shown to reduce the incidences of apnea and hypopnea episodes when compared to the preoperative baseline. CPAP is associated with improved ventilation in postoperative OSA patient and also it has shown reduced hospital stay [95–97].

Patients who receive long-acting opioids should be monitored closely and may need high dependency unit admission for postoperative monitoring. Indications for obese patients with OSA for HDU or ICU admission are preexisting co-morbidities, limited functional capacity, major surgery, poorly controlled OSA requiring systemic opioids. The patient should be discharged to the unmonitored settings only when adequate oxygen saturation is maintained to baseline level on room air and with no more risk of respiratory depression (apnea or hypopnea) that can be determined ideally when the patient is asleep [91].

10. Recommendations from guidelines in obese patients with OSA

High-risk OSA patients should be managed by a dedicated specialized anesthesia team. Regional anesthetic technique or nonopioids analgesics should be used to reduce the need for systemic opioids. Meticulous monitoring is required when sedatives and opioids are used in suspected or OSA patients due to high risk of respiratory depression. Even HDU or ICU admission for monitoring could be considered if obesity is associated with other co-morbidities. OSA and its complications should be anticipated in obese patient. Postoperative use of supplemental oxygen is recommended as it reduces the incidence of hypoxemic episodes, in addition to CPAP or NIPPV, that could relieve the upper airway obstruction.

Author details

Sayed Rahman[1], Ahmed Zaghw[2]*, Osama Elazzouny[2], Dhari Almenshid[2], Mustafa Rezk[2], Mohammed Azizuddin Imran[3] and Malek Alali[2]

*Address all correspondence to: ahmedzaghw@gmail.com

1 John H. Stroger Jr. Hospital of Cook County, Chicago, IL, USA

2 Hamad Medical Corporation, Doha, Qatar

3 Women's Wellness and Research Center, Doha, Qatar

References

[1] WHO. Overweight and obesity. WHO; 2017

[2] Punjabi NM, Sorkin JD, Katzel LI, Goldberg AP, Schwartz AR, Smith PL. Sleep-disordered breathing and insulin resistance in middle-aged and overweight men. American Journal of Respiratory and Critical Care Medicine. 2002 Mar 1;**165**(5):677-682

[3] Peppard PE, Young T, Palta M, Dempsey J, Skatrud J. Longitudinal study of moderate weight change and sleep-disordered breathing. Journal of the American Medical Association. 2000 Dec 20;**284**(23):3015-3021

[4] Garvey WT, Mechanick JI, Brett EM, Garber AJ, Hurley DL, Jastreboff AM, et al. American Association of Clinical Endocrinologists and American College of Endocrinology comprehensive clinical practice guidelines for medical care of patients with obesity. Endocrine Practice. 2016 Jul;**22** Suppl 3:1-203

[5] Epstein LJ, Kristo D, Strollo PJ, Friedman N, Malhotra A, Patil SP, et al. Clinical guideline for the evaluation, management and long-term care of obstructive sleep apnea in adults. Journal of Clinical Sleep Medicine. 2009 Jun 15;**5**(3):263-276

[6] Hiestand DM, Britz P, Goldman M, Phillips B. Prevalence of symptoms and risk of sleep apnea in the US population: Results from the national sleep foundation sleep in America 2005 poll. Chest. 2006 Sep;**130**(3):780-786

[7] Sateia MJ. International classification of sleep disorders-third edition: Highlights and modifications. Chest. 2014 Nov;**146**(5):1387-1394

[8] Reichmuth KJ, Austin D, Skatrud JB, Young T. Association of sleep apnea and type II diabetes: A population-based study. American Journal of Respiratory and Critical Care Medicine. 2005 Dec 15;**172**(12):1590-1595

[9] Peppard PE, Young T, Palta M, Skatrud J. Prospective study of the association between sleep-disordered breathing and hypertension. The New England Journal of Medicine. 2000 May 11;**342**(19):1378-1384

[10] Punjabi NM, Caffo BS, Goodwin JL, Gottlieb DJ, Newman AB, O'Connor GT, et al. Sleep-disordered breathing and mortality: A prospective cohort study. Patel A, editor. PLoS Medicine. 2009 Aug 18;**6**(8):e1000132

[11] Hermann DM, Bassetti CL. Role of sleep-disordered breathing and sleep-wake disturbances for stroke and stroke recovery. Neurology. 2016 Sep 27;**87**(13):1407-1416

[12] Marshall NS, Wong KKH, Liu PY, Cullen SRJ, Knuiman MW, Grunstein RR. Sleep apnea as an independent risk factor for all-cause mortality: The Busselton health study. Sleep. 2008 Aug;**31**(8):1079-1085

[13] Redline S, Tishler PV, Tosteson TD, Williamson J, Kump K, Browner I, et al. The familial aggregation of obstructive sleep apnea. American Journal of Respiratory and Critical Care Medicine. 1995 Mar;**151**(3 Pt 1):682-687

[14] Chi L, Comyn F-L, Mitra N, Reilly MP, Wan F, Maislin G, et al. Identification of craniofacial risk factors for obstructive sleep apnoea using three-dimensional MRI. The European Respiratory Journal. 2011 Aug 1;**38**(2):348-358

[15] Haba-Rubio J, Sforza E, Weiss T, Schröder C, Krieger J. Effect of CPAP treatment on inspiratory arousal threshold during NREM sleep in OSAS. Sleep & Breathing. 2005 Mar; **9**(1):12-19

[16] Rowley JA, Zahn BR, Babcock MA, Badr MS. The effect of rapid eye movement (REM) sleep on upper airway mechanics in normal human subjects. The Journal of Physiology. 1998 Aug 1;**510**(Pt 3):963-976

[17] Rowley JA, Sanders CS, Zahn BR, Badr MS. Gender differences in upper airway compliance during NREM sleep: Role of neck circumference. Journal of Applied Physiology. 2002 Jun;**92**(6):2535-2541

[18] Badr MS, Skatrud JB, Dempsey JA, Begle RL. Effect of mechanical loading on expiratory and inspiratory muscle activity during NREM sleep. Journal of Applied Physiology. 1990 Mar;**68**(3):1195-1202

[19] Gleeson K, Zwillich CW, White DP. The influence of increasing ventilatory effort on arousal from sleep. The American Review of Respiratory Disease. 1990 Aug;**142**(2):295-300

[20] Jordan AS, Eckert DJ, Wellman A, Trinder JA, Malhotra A, White DP. Termination of respiratory events with and without cortical arousal in obstructive sleep apnea. American Journal of Respiratory and Critical Care Medicine. 2011 Nov 15;**184**(10):1183-1191

[21] Wilkinson V, Malhotra A, Nicholas CL, Worsnop C, Jordan AS, Butler JE, et al. Discharge patterns of human genioglossus motor units during arousal from sleep. Sleep. 2010 Mar; **33**(3):379-387

[22] Walker JM, Farney RJ, Rhondeau SM, Boyle KM, Valentine K, Cloward TV, et al. Chronic opioid use is a risk factor for the development of central sleep apnea and ataxic breathing. Journal of Clinical Sleep Medicine. 2007 Aug 15;**3**(5):455-461

[23] Sharkey KM, Kurth ME, Anderson BJ, Corso RP, Millman RP, Stein MD. Obstructive sleep apnea is more common than central sleep apnea in methadone maintenance patients with subjective sleep complaints. Drug and Alcohol Dependence. 2010 Apr 1;**108**(1–2):77-83

[24] Chung F, Liao P, Elsaid H, Shapiro CM, Kang W. Factors associated with postoperative exacerbation of sleep-disordered breathing. Anesthesiology. 2014 Feb;**120**(2):299-311

[25] Boostani R, Rezaeitalab F, Pourmokhtari B, Ghahremani A. Sleep apnea headaches. Reviews in Clinical Medicine. 2016 Jan 1;**3**(1):1-3

[26] Somers VK, White DP, Amin R, Abraham WT, Costa F, Culebras A, et al. Sleep apnea and cardiovascular disease: An American Heart Association/American College of Cardiology foundation scientific statement from the American Heart Association Council for High Blood Pressure Research Professional Education Committee, Council on Clinical Cardiology, Stroke Council, and Council On Cardiovascular Nursing. In collaboration with the

National Heart, Lung, and Blood Institute National Center on sleep disorders research (National Institutes of Health). Circulation. 2008 Sep 2;**118**(10):1080-1111

[27] Kumar DS, Valenzuela D, Kozak FK, Ludemann JP, Moxham JP, Lea J, et al. The reliability of clinical tonsil size grading in children. JAMA Otolaryngology. Head & Neck Surgery. 2014 Nov 1;**140**(11):1034-1037

[28] Celebi S, Tepe C, Yelken K, Celik O. Efficacy of dexpanthenol for pediatric post-tonsillectomy pain and wound healing. The Annals of Otology, Rhinology, and Laryngology. 2013 Jul;**122**(7): 464-467

[29] Troell RJ, Powell NB, Riley RW, Li KK, Guilleminault C. Comparison of postoperative pain between laser-assisted uvulopalatoplasty, uvulopalatopharyngoplasty, and radiofrequency volumetric tissue reduction of the palate. Otolaryngology and Head and Neck Surgery. 2000 Mar;**122**(3):402-409

[30] Ogunnaike BO, Jones SB, Jones DB, Provost D, Whitten CW. Anesthetic considerations for bariatric surgery. Anesthesia and Analgesia. 2002 Dec;**95**(6):1793-1805

[31] Brown KA, Laferrière A, Lakheeram I, Moss IR. Recurrent hypoxemia in children is associated with increased analgesic sensitivity to opiates. Anesthesiology. 2006 Oct;**105**(4):665-669

[32] Wu J, Li P, Wu X, Chen W. Chronic intermittent hypoxia decreases pain sensitivity and increases the expression of HIF1α and opioid receptors in experimental rats. Sleep & Breathing. 2015 May 10;**19**(2):561-568

[33] Ferguson LM, Drummond GB. Acute effects of fentanyl on breathing pattern in anaesthetized subjects. British Journal of Anaesthesia. 2006 Mar;**96**(3):384-390

[34] Overdyk FJ, Hillman DR. Opioid modeling of central respiratory drive must take upper airway obstruction into account. Anesthesiology. 2011 Jan;**114**(1):219-220 author reply 220-1

[35] Benyamin R, Trescot AM, Datta S, Buenaventura R, Adlaka R, Sehgal N, et al. Opioid complications and side effects. Pain Physician. 2008 Mar;**11**(2 Suppl):S105-S120

[36] Hartwell EE, Pfeifer JG, McCauley JL, Moran-Santa Maria M, Back SE. Sleep disturbances and pain among individuals with prescription opioid dependence. Addictive Behaviors. 2014 Oct;**39**(10):1537-1542

[37] DeSouza G, Lewis MC, TerRiet MF. Severe bradycardia after remifentanil. Anesthesiology. 1997 Oct;**87**(4):1019-1020

[38] Latta KS, Ginsberg B, Barkin RL. Meperidine: a critical review. American Journal of Therapeutics;**9**(1):53-68

[39] Chen A, Ashburn MA. Cardiac effects of opioid therapy. Pain Medicine. 2015 Oct 1;**16** Suppl 1:S27-S31

[40] Reeder MK, Goldman MD, Loh L, Muir AD, Casey KR, Lehane JR. Late postoperative nocturnal dips in oxygen saturation in patients undergoing major abdominal vascular

surgery. Predictive value of pre-operative overnight pulse oximetry. Anaesthesia. 1992 Feb;**47**(2):110-115

[41] Madan AK, Ternovits CA, Speck KE, Tichansky DS. Inpatient pain medication requirements after laparoscopic gastric bypass. Obesity Surgery;**15**(6):778-781

[42] Govindarajan R, Ghosh B, Sathyamoorthy MK, Kodali NS, Raza A, Aronsohn J, et al. Efficacy of ketorolac in lieu of narcotics in the operative management of laparoscopic surgery for morbid obesity. Surgery for Obesity and Related Diseases;**1**(6):530-535 discussion 535-6

[43] Ingrasciotta Y, Sultana J, Giorgianni F, Fontana A, Santangelo A, Tari DU, et al. Association of individual non-steroidal anti-inflammatory drugs and chronic kidney disease: A population-based case control study. Seguro AC, editor. PLoS One. 2015 Apr 16;**10**(4):e0122899

[44] Lipworth L, Abdel-Kader K, Morse J, Stewart TG, Kabagambe EK, Parr SK, et al. High prevalence of non-steroidal anti-inflammatory drug use among acute kidney injury survivors in the southern community cohort study. BMC Nephrology. 2016;**17**(1):189

[45] Cotter JT, Nielsen KC, Guller U, Steele SM, Klein SM, Greengrass RA, et al. Increased body mass index and ASA physical status IV are risk factors for block failure in ambulatory surgery: An analysis of 9,342 blocks. Canadian Journal of Anaesthesia. 2004 Oct;**51**(8): 810-816

[46] Franco CD, Gloss FJ, Voronov G, Tyler SG, Stojiljkovic LS. Supraclavicular block in the obese population: An analysis of 2020 blocks. Anesthesia and Analgesia. 2006 Apr;**102**(4): 1252-1254

[47] Remy C, Marret E, Bonnet F. Effects of acetaminophen on morphine side-effects and consumption after major surgery: Meta-analysis of randomized controlled trials. British Journal of Anaesthesia. 2005 Apr;**94**(4):505-513

[48] Song K, Melroy MJ, Whipple OC. Optimizing multimodal analgesia with intravenous acetaminophen and opioids in postoperative bariatric patients. Pharmacotherapy. 2014 Dec;**34** Suppl 1:14S-21S

[49] Ryu J-H, Kang M-H, Park K-S, Do S-H. Effects of magnesium sulphate on intraoperative anaesthetic requirements and postoperative analgesia in gynaecology patients receiving total intravenous anaesthesia. British Journal of Anaesthesia. 2008 Mar;**100**(3):397-403

[50] Hassani V, Pazouki A, Nikoubakht N, Chaichian S, Sayarifard A, Shakib KA. The effect of gabapentin on reducing pain after laparoscopic gastric bypass surgery in patients with morbid obesity: A randomized clinical trial. Anesthesiology and Pain Medicine. 2015 Feb 1; **5**(1):e22372

[51] Eipe N, Penning J. Postoperative respiratory depression with pregabalin: A case series and a preoperative decision algorithm. Pain Research & Management;**16**(5):353-356

[52] Bidaki R, Sadeghi Z, Shafizadegan S, Sadeghi A, Khalili B, Haghshenas A, et al. Gabapentin induces edema, hyperesthesia and scaling in a depressed patient; a diagnostic challenge. Advanced Biomedical Research. 2016;**5**(1):1

[53] Blaudszun G, Lysakowski C, Elia N, Tramèr MR. Effect of perioperative systemic α2 agonists on postoperative morphine consumption and pain intensity: Systematic review and meta-analysis of randomized controlled trials. Anesthesiology. 2012 Jun;**116**(6): 1312-1322

[54] Bamgbade OA, Alfa JA. Dexmedetomidine anaesthesia for patients with obstructive sleep apnoea undergoing bariatric surgery. European Journal of Anaesthesiology. 2009 Feb; **26**(2):176-177

[55] Feld JM, Hoffman WE, Stechert MM, Hoffman IW, Ananda RC. Fentanyl or dexmedetomidine combined with desflurane for bariatric surgery. Journal of Clinical Anesthesia. 2006 Feb;**18**(1):24-28

[56] Singh PM, Panwar R, Borle A, Mulier JP, Sinha A, Goudra B. Perioperative analgesic profile of dexmedetomidine infusions in morbidly obese undergoing bariatric surgery: A meta-analysis and trial sequential analysis. Surgery for Obesity and Related Diseases. 2017 Aug;**13**(8):1434-1446

[57] Kibler LE, Gazes PC. Effect of clonidine on atrioventricular conduction. Journal of the American Medical Association. 1977 Oct;**238**(18):1930-1932

[58] Sollazzi L, Modesti C, Vitale F, Sacco T, Ciocchetti P, Idra AS, et al. Preinductive use of clonidine and ketamine improves recovery and reduces postoperative pain after bariatric surgery. Surgery for Obesity and Related Diseases. 2009 Jan;**5**(1):67-71

[59] Feld JM, Laurito CE, Beckerman M, Vincent J, Hoffman WE. Non-opioid analgesia improves pain relief and decreases sedation after gastric bypass surgery. Canadian Journal of Anaesthesia. 2003 Apr;**50**(4):336-341

[60] Nossaman VE, Ramadhyani U, Kadowitz PJ, Nossaman BD. Advances in perioperative pain management: Use of medications with dual analgesic mechanisms, tramadol & tapentadol. Anesthesiology Clinics. 2010 Dec;**28**(4):647-666

[61] Chou R, Gordon DB, de Leon-Casasola OA, Rosenberg JM, Bickler S, Brennan T, et al. Management of Postoperative Pain: A clinical practice guideline from the American Pain Society, the American Society of Regional Anesthesia and Pain Medicine, and the American Society of Anesthesiologists' Committee on Regional Anesthesia, Executive Committee, and Administrative Council. The Journal of Pain. 2016 Feb;**17**(2):131-157

[62] Ziemann-Gimmel P, Hensel P, Koppman J, Marema R. Multimodal analgesia reduces narcotic requirements and antiemetic rescue medication in laparoscopic Roux-en-Y gastric bypass surgery. Surgery for Obesity and Related Diseases. 2013 Nov;**9**(6):975-980

[63] Abdallah FW, Chan VW, Brull R. Transversus abdominis plane block: A systematic review. Regional Anesthesia and Pain Medicine. 2012;**37**(2):193-209

[64] De Oliveira GS, Duncan K, Fitzgerald P, Nader A, Gould RW, McCarthy RJ. Systemic lidocaine to improve quality of recovery after laparoscopic bariatric surgery: A randomized double-blinded placebo-controlled trial. Obesity Surgery. 2014 Feb 15;**24**(2):212-218

[65] Hadzic A, Williams BA, Karaca PE, Hobeika P, Unis G, Dermksian J, et al. For outpatient rotator cuff surgery, nerve block anesthesia provides superior same-day recovery over general anesthesia. Anesthesiology. 2005 May;**102**(5):1001-1007

[66] Kaw R, Pasupuleti V, Walker E, Ramaswamy A, Foldvary-Schafer N. Postoperative complications in patients with obstructive sleep apnea. Chest. 2012 Feb;**141**(2):436-441

[67] Gupta RM, Parvizi J, Hanssen AD, Gay PC. Postoperative complications in patients with obstructive sleep apnea syndrome undergoing hip or knee replacement: A case-control study. Mayo Clinic Proceedings. 2001 Sep;**76**(9):897-905

[68] Block BM, Liu SS, Rowlingson AJ, Cowan AR, Cowan JA, Wu CL. Efficacy of postoperative epidural analgesia: A meta-analysis. Journal of the American Medical Association. 2003 Nov 12;**290**(18):2455-2463

[69] Richman JM, Liu SS, Courpas G, Wong R, Rowlingson AJ, McGready J, et al. Does continuous peripheral nerve block provide superior pain control to opioids? A meta-analysis. Anesthesia and Analgesia. 2006 Jan;**102**(1):248-257

[70] Liu SS, Wu CL. The effect of analgesic technique on postoperative patient-reported outcomes including analgesia: A systematic review. Anesthesia and Analgesia. 2007 Sep;**105**(3): 789-808

[71] Liu SS, Wu CL. Effect of postoperative analgesia on major postoperative complications: A systematic update of the evidence. Anesthesia and Analgesia. 2007 Mar;**104**(3):689-702

[72] Kapala M, Meterissian S, Schricker T. Neuraxial anesthesia and intraoperative bilevel positive airway pressure in a patient with severe chronic obstructive pulmonary disease and obstructive sleep apnea undergoing elective sigmoid resection. Regional Anesthesia and Pain Medicine. 2009 Jan;**34**(1):69-71

[73] Smetana GW. Postoperative pulmonary complications: An update on risk assessment and reduction. Cleveland Clinic Journal of Medicine. 2009 Nov 1;**76**Suppl 4:S60-S65

[74] von Ungern-Sternberg BS, Regli A, Reber A, Schneider MC. Effect of obesity and thoracic epidural analgesia on perioperative spirometry. British Journal of Anaesthesia. 2005 Jan;**94**(1): 121-127

[75] Taivainen T, Tuominen M, Rosenberg PH. Influence of obesity on the spread of spinal analgesia after injection of plain 0.5% bupivacaine at the L3-4 or L4-5 interspace. British Journal of Anaesthesia. 1990 May;**64**(5):542-546

[76] Ostermeier AM, Roizen MF, Hautkappe M, Klock PA, Klafta JM. Three sudden postoperative respiratory arrests associated with epidural opioids in patients with sleep apnea. Anesthesia and Analgesia. 1997 Aug;**85**(2):452-460

[77] Ellinas EH, Eastwood DC, Patel SN, Maitra-D'Cruze AM, Ebert TJ. The effect of obesity on neuraxial technique difficulty in pregnant patients: A prospective, observational study. Anesthesia and Analgesia. 2009 Oct;**109**(4):1225-1231

[78] Perlas A, Chaparro LE, Chin KJ. Lumbar Neuraxial ultrasound for spinal and epidural anesthesia: A systematic review and meta-analysis. Regional Anesthesia and Pain Medicine. 2016;**41**(2):251-260

[79] Al-Nasser B. Review of interscalene block for postoperative analgesia after shoulder surgery in obese patients. Acta Anaesthesiologica Taiwanica. 2012 Mar;**50**(1):29-34

[80] Naja ZM, Naccache N, Ziade F, El-Rajab M, Itani T, Baraka A. Multilevel nerve stimulator-guided paravertebral block as a sole anesthetic technique for breast cancer surgery in morbidly obese patients. Journal of Anesthesia. 2011 Oct 12;**25**(5):760-764

[81] Dahl JB, Møiniche S. Pre-emptive analgesia. British Medical Bulletin. 2004;**71**:13-27

[82] Grass JA. Patient-controlled analgesia. Anesthesia and Analgesia. 2005 Nov;**101**(5 Suppl): S44-S61

[83] Sherwinter DA, Ghaznavi AM, Spinner D, Savel RH, Macura JM, Adler H. Continuous infusion of intraperitoneal bupivacaine after laparoscopic surgery: A randomized controlled trial. Obesity Surgery. 2008 Dec 22;**18**(12):1581-1586

[84] Forastiere E, Sofra M, Giannarelli D, Fabrizi L, Simone G. Effectiveness of continuous wound infusion of 0.5% ropivacaine by On-Q pain relief system for postoperative pain management after open nephrectomy. British Journal of Anaesthesia. 2008 Dec;**101**(6): 841-847

[85] Lloret-Linares C, Lopes A, Declèves X, Serrie A, Mouly S, Bergmann J-F, et al. Challenges in the optimisation of post-operative pain management with opioids in obese patients: A literature review. Obesity Surgery. 2013 Sep 23;**23**(9):1458-1475

[86] Malanga GA, Yan N, Stark J. Mechanisms and efficacy of heat and cold therapies for musculoskeletal injury. Postgraduate Medicine. 2015 Jan;**127**(1):57-65

[87] Alimi D, Rubino C, Pichard-Léandri E, Fermand-Brulé S, Dubreuil-Lemaire M-L, Hill C. Analgesic effect of auricular acupuncture for cancer pain: A randomized, blinded, controlled trial. Journal of Clinical Oncology. 2003 Nov 15;**21**(22):4120-4126

[88] American Society of Anesthesiologists Task Force on Postanesthetic Care. Practice guidelines for postanesthetic care: A report by the American Society of Anesthesiologists Task Force on Postanesthetic care. Anesthesiology. 2002 Mar;**96**(3):742-752

[89] Prathanvanich P, Chand B. The role of capnography during upper endoscopy in morbidly obese patients: A prospective study. Surgery for Obesity and Related Diseases. 2015 Jan; **11**(1):193-198

[90] Krauss B, Hess DR. Capnography for procedural sedation and analgesia in the emergency department. Annals of Emergency Medicine. 2007 Aug;**50**(2):172-181

[91] American Society of Anesthesiologists Task Force on Perioperative Management of patients with obstructive sleep apnea. Practice guidelines for the perioperative management of patients with obstructive sleep apnea: An updated report by the American Society

of Anesthesiologists Task Force on perioperative management of patients with obstructive sleep apnea. Anesthesiology. 2014 Feb;**120**(2):268-286

[92] Members of the Working Party CE, Nightingale CE, Margarson MP, Shearer E, Redman JW, Lucas DN, et al. Peri-operative management of the obese surgical patient 2015: Association of Anaesthetists of Great Britain and Ireland Society for Obesity and Bariatric Anaesthesia. Anaesthesia. 2015 Jul;**70**(7):859-876

[93] Biro P, Kaplan V, Bloch KE. Anesthetic management of a patient with obstructive sleep apnea syndrome and difficult airway access. Journal of Clinical Anesthesia. 1995 Aug;**7**(5): 417-421

[94] Chung F, Memtsoudis SG, Ramachandran SK, Nagappa M, Opperer M, Cozowicz C, et al. Society of Anesthesia and Sleep Medicine Guidelines on preoperative screening and assessment of adult patients with obstructive sleep apnea. Anesthesia and Analgesia. 2016 Aug;**123**(2):452-473

[95] Nagappa M, Mokhlesi B, Wong J, Wong DT, Kaw R, Chung F. The effects of continuous positive airway pressure on postoperative outcomes in obstructive sleep apnea patients undergoing surgery: A systematic review and meta-analysis. Anesthesia and Analgesia. 2015 May;**120**(5):1013-1023

[96] Gross JB, Bachenberg KL, Benumof JL, Caplan RA, Connis RT, Coté CJ, et al. Practice guidelines for the perioperative management of patients with obstructive sleep apnea: A report by the American Society of Anesthesiologists Task Force on perioperative management of patients with obstructive sleep apnea. Anesthesiology. 2006 May;**104**(5):1081-1093 quiz 1117-8

[97] Neligan PJ, Malhotra G, Fraser M, Williams N, Greenblatt EP, Cereda M, et al. Continuous positive airway pressure via the Boussignac system immediately after extubation improves lung function in morbidly obese patients with obstructive sleep apnea undergoing laparoscopic bariatric surgery. Anesthesiology. 2009 Apr;**110**(4):878-884